MIXING MEDICINES

INTOXICATING HISTORIES

Series Editors: Virginia Berridge and Erika Dyck

Whether on the street, off the shelf, or over the pharmacy counter, interactions with drugs and alcohol are shaped by contested ideas about addiction, healing, pleasure, and vice and their social dimensions. Books in this series explore how people around the world have consumed, created, traded, and regulated psychoactive substances throughout history. The series connects research on legal and illegal drugs and alcohol with diverse areas of historical inquiry, including the histories of medicine, pharmacy, consumption, trade, law, social policy, and popular culture. Its reach is global and includes scholarship on all periods. Intoxicating Histories aims to link these different pasts as well as to inform the present by providing a firmer grasp on contemporary debates and policy issues. We welcome books, whether scholarly monographs or shorter texts for a broad audience focusing on a particular phenomenon or substance, that alter the state of knowledge.

1 Taming Cannabis
Drugs and Empire in Nineteenth-Century France
David A. Guba, Jr

2 Cigarette Nation
Business, Health, and Canadian Smokers, 1930–1975
Daniel J. Robinson

3 Remedicalising Cannabis
Science, Industry, and Drug Policy
Suzanne Taylor

4 Mixing Medicines
The Global Drug Trade and Early Modern Russia
Clare Griffin

Mixing Medicines

The Global Drug Trade and Early Modern Russia

CLARE GRIFFIN

McGill-Queen's University Press
Montreal & Kingston . London . Chicago

ISBN 978-0-2280-1193-4 (cloth)
ISBN 978-0-2280-1194-1 (paper)
ISBN 978-0-2280-1283-2 (ePDF)
ISBN 978-0-2280-1284-9 (ePUB)
ISBN 978-0-2280-1476-8 (OA)

Legal deposit third quarter 2022
Bibliothèque nationale du Québec

The open access edition of this book was funded by the Wellcome Trust.

Library and Archives Canada Cataloguing in Publication

Title: Mixing medicines : the global drug trade and early modern Russia / Clare Griffin.
Names: Griffin, Clare, author.
Series: Intoxicating histories ; 4.
Description: Series statement: Intoxicating histories ; 4 | Includes bibliographical references and index.
Identifiers: Canadiana (print) 2022019906x | Canadiana (ebook) 20220199108 | ISBN 9780228011941 (paper) | ISBN 9780228011934 (cloth) | ISBN 9780228012832 (ePDF) | ISBN 9780228012849 (ePUB) | ISBN 9780228014768 (OA)
Subjects: LCSH: Materia medica—Russia—History. | LCSH: Drugs—Russia—History.
Classification: LCC RS177.R9 G75 2022 | DDC 615.3/210947—dc23

This book was typeset by True to Type in 11.5/14 Arno Pro

To Everyone Who Helped

Всем, кто помог

Contents

Acknowledgments

Writing the acknowledgments is simultaneously the nicest and the scariest part of completing this book. This work would never have been finished without the patience and kindness of innumerable people. I can only hope I have remembered all of you and spoken of you as warmly as I feel.

This book has been greatly improved by the patient work of many hands. I thank my editor Kyla Madden, two anonymous peer reviewers, and everyone at McGill-Queen's University Press, as well as Amberle Sherman, Audra Wolfe, Ramey Moore, and Oksana Vynnyk, all of whom did so much to make this book as good as it could be. Thanks also to the Eurasian Studies reading group at Nazarbayev University; Lauren Kassell and her Premodern Medicine reading group at Cambridge; Alisha Rankin, Jennifer Rampling, Lorraine Daston, and her group at the Max Planck Institute for the History of Science (MPIWG), Berlin; Christopher Nicholson; and everyone else who so kindly offered their thoughts on drafts of this book.

I am indebted to the staff of many libraries and archives, without whose expertise I would have been lost. The libraries and archives of Moscow are some of my favourite places in the world, and I have been lucky to work with many other wonderful collections as well. My thanks to the staff of the Nazarbayev University Library here in Nur-Sultan; the MPIWG library in Berlin; Stadsarchief Amsterdam; the National Library of Russia and Library of the Academy of Sciences in St Petersburg; and the Russian State Library and State Historical Museum in Moscow. Most of all, my very deepest thanks to the wonderful people and cats of the Russian State Archive of Ancient Documents, Moscow – my home away from home for so many months – for your patience and kindness in helping me find, copy, and understand the materials I rely upon in this book.

I am hugely grateful to the entirety of the School of Slavonic and East European Studies, University College London, my three-time alma mater, for keeping me around for so long, and in particular to Faith Wigzell, who was the first person to tell me I could be good at this; to my PhD supervisors Sergei Bogatyrev, Harold J. Cook, and Martyn Rady; and to my PhD examiners, the Simons Dixon and Franklin.

I have been lucky enough to have had wonderful colleagues along the way. *Astanchane* current and former Meiramgul Kussainova; David Moon; Zbig Wojnowski; my officemate Curtis Murphy and the rest of the HPRS team; Zhanar Jampeissova; and many other kind *sobesedniki* and excellent colleagues. During my time in Berlin I benefited from the kindness and insights of Lorraine Daston and Dagmar Schäfer and the many lovely people in their departments, as well as the company of Tul'si Bhambry, Sabine Dumschat, Jacob Gaboury, Markham J. Geller and Florentina Badalanova-Geller, Alexei Evstratov and Kirill Ospovat, Hans-Uwe Lammel, and Lukas Macher. In Moscow I have enjoyed the hospitality and warmth of so many who were ready and willing to welcome the strange foreign lady, including Evgenii V. Akel'ev, Aleksandra B. Ippolitova, Sergei M. Kashtanov, Kirill S. Khudin, Juli Levickaja, Boris N. Morozov, Rem A. Simonov, Elena B. Smilianskaia, Andrei L. Toporkov, Andrei V. Topychkanov, Konstantin Yu. Jerusalimskii, and many others. I am grateful also to my fellow explorers of Muscovy from afar: Eve Levin; Valerie Kivelson; Matthew P. Romaniello; as well as Alison Smith and Tricia Starks, whom I will forever think of as honorary Muscovite historians; as well as to my other wonderful colleagues Sanjoy Bhattacharya, Anna Graber, Rachel Koroloff, Simon Werrett, Audra Yoder, and many more besides. Thanks also to my fellow explorers of the arcane roadways of the early modern drugs trade: Samir Boumedienne, Pratik Chakrabarti, Harun Küçük, Carla Nappi, Valentina Pugliano, Emma Spary, Michael Stanley-Baker, Jan Willem Veluwenkamp, and Patrick Wallis. Your work has made mine better.

To my academic sisters Layla AbdelRahim, Soha Bayoumi, Katia Bowers, Emma Hagström-Molin, Eleanor Janega, Sydney Morrow, Aparna Nair, Lisa Onaga, and Jaya Remond, thank you for always understanding. To those wise enough to avoid the academic maelstrom, Charlotte Jones and Victoria Reynolds-O'Brien, thank you for making the effort to understand what it possibly could be that I get up to. And to Erika L. Milam and Michael D. Gordin, tireless adopters of waifs and strays everywhere, I could never have done this without you.

This book was possible because of the support and funding of several institutions. I first began my voyage through the murky waters of the early modern medical drugs trade as a Wellcome Trust Research Fellow (grant no. 101554/Z/13/Z) at the Department of History and Philosophy of Science, University of Cambridge, then journeyed onwards to the Max Planck Institute for the History of Science, Berlin, to join Elaine Leong's "Reading and Writing Nature in Early Modern Europe" MPG Minerva Research Group, before making landfall at my present location, Nazarbayev University. I thank all these institutions and organizations for giving me the opportunity to undertake, and finally to finish, this work.

Last, but as they say, nowhere near least, I thank Simon, as well as Zarya and Whiskey, the tiniest of monsters, for supporting me through this, and reminding me that there are more things in heaven and earth than this book manuscript.

MIXING MEDICINES

Introduction

In 1664, the British physician Samuel Collins sat down in Moscow to write a report in Latin for his Russian masters. One of a number of Western European medical practitioners vital to the Apothecary Chancery, the Muscovite palace medical department, writing such texts on the orders of Russian administrators was a key part of Collins's job; once he – or one of his fellow physicians – had written the text in Latin, it was then translated into Chancery Russian, all the better to be consumed by the Russian elite.[1] On this occasion, the narrative was one of global *materia medica,* told through stereotypes of the peoples of the early modern world.

> There are in creation peoples whose lives, customs, and thoughts are only of medical drugs; not one nation appears so unthoughtful as to – whether by accident or out of certain unavoidable necessities – fail to acquire and put into use drugs whose virtues are hidden from others. Brazilian tribes in America, naked and illiterate, nevertheless have their own, not unworthy medicines, having brought into use the tree sassafras, guaiacum, jalap, and many other plants of unusual powers. Miracles are told of the Chinese doctors, by whose art serious diseases are driven away without venesection or bloodletting, and with only the use of herbal simples of their own creation. Indians drive out illnesses with the steam from boiling herbs with special properties, not with the oils that slaves apply and gently scrape from nobles by hand, to which habit the nobles are so accustomed that they cannot sleep without it. Every year the great Mogul emperor of the Indians would elevate one of his doctors, and that doctor would hold forth his judgments on the excess or deficits of the emperor's body. And

> there is an ancient custom amongst the Persians, to which Daniel may have referred to in his Prophecy in the presence of King Belshazzar. Arabs, Chaldeans, Greeks, Latins, allow any medicines (judged in their eyes to be healthy).[2]

This text, with its presentation of medical practitioners and their practices from around the early modern global world, reflects key aspects of early modern Russian medical culture. In documents from the sixteenth, seventeenth, and early eighteenth centuries, there is a notable focus on *materia medica* as both useful and potentially dangerous. The difference between a medicine consumed to help the human body and a potion that once consumed would harm it was never as significant as people wished it to be. Moreover, those objects can be traced through early modern trading networks to a wide range of geographical origins. Just as Collins here invokes the medical practices of both the Americas and East Asia, prescriptions written by him and his colleagues brought together ingredients from those far-flung locations, and many others besides. This material then points us in a very specific direction: to an examination of the *materia medica* of early modern Russia as a history of global connections shaping the practice of medicine.

MATERIA MEDICA AS MATERIAL CULTURE

The paradox of early modern Russian medical records is that we have both notable survivals and problematic absences. In particular for the seventeenth century, we have sometimes day-by-day accounts of the specific medicaments prescribed to the tsar, a kind of detailed elite pharmacy record that has rarely survived in other locations. We also have lists of imports, inventories from the court medical department, reports of various kinds and a number of pharmacy texts. What we often lack are explanatory documents. In the case of most prescriptions, we are given the name of the patient, the name of the prescribing physician and/or the apothecary creating the medicine, and the list of ingredients. No mention of the disease treated. No mention of the medical theory underpinning diagnosis and cure. The clearest point emerging from these documents is the materials of pharmacy practice.

These facts fundamentally shape the questions we can ask here, and take us in a useful direction for the history and science and medicine.

Looking at materials gives us a more tactile history than considering theory texts. We can move from theory – what should happen – to practice – what did happen. However, such tactile histories are hampered by the fact that too often the actual materials of historical science and medicine were destroyed or lost. Yet their absence should not mean that we should ignore them; they are simply too important a part of that history to leave aside. Here, we can circumvent this issue by looking at documents about materials. This does not give us the same view of historical scientific and medical practices as having the actual materials would, but it does give us a vital window onto that history. We can then ask, what can these *materia medica* documents tell us about early modern medicine? And in particular, what does the specific interest in medical drugs tell us about material culture and the history of science and medicine?

Histories of pharmacy are numerous and are often focused on such a set of documents, where happenstance archival survivals allow us to see the everyday practices of a particular time and place. He Bian's *Know Your Remedies* looks at the remarkable variety of documents on pharmacy shops in early modern China.[3] Recent attention has been paid to the *pharmacopoeia* as a genre of text, notably the edited volume *Drugs on the Page*, focusing on those kinds of texts in the early modern Atlantic world.[4] Major cities have often been the subject of such studies, such as Leigh Chipman's on Mamluk Cairo, Hjalmar Fors's work on Stockholm, Linda A. Newson's on Colonial Lima, and James Shaw and Florence Welch's work on Renaissance Florence.[5] Histories of early modern science and medicine, including histories of pharmacy, rarely consider the Russian Empire, despite its being a major power. In part, this book is in this tradition of histories of pharmacy in major cities, being the first book devoted to pharmacy in early modern Moscow.

The immediate locale of the Apothecary Chancery records is Moscow; their importance goes substantially beyond those city limits. Collins's account of the *materia medica* of the early modern world is typical for these documents. Prescriptions from the 1580s show the use of European, African, and Asian materials. After 1600, the department imported an increasing range of American ingredients. This then is also a story of the early modern global drugs trade. There is now a substantial historiography on this topic, with particular focus on the Atlantic world. Works by Samir Boumedienne, Harold J. Cook, Teresa Huguet-Termes, Patrick Wallis, Timothy Walker, have all given vital insight into how

American materials were appropriated from Indigenous communities, transported across the Atlantic, and incorporated into Western European medicine.[6] Similarly, much attention has been devoted to the circulation of objects, texts, and ideas between East Asia and Western Europe.[7] We know much about the initial stages of acquiring drugs, and of middlemen moving drugs around.

American medical ingredients did not stop in Western Europe. Stephanie Gänger has shown that by the eighteenth century a number of those materials were being sold and used in multiple locations across Afro-Eurasia.[8] This aspect of the Atlantic exchange is under-researched. American products were only worth the huge costs and great dangers of acquiring and transporting them if someone would buy them. Yet we do not always have the records to see the end use of these products, such a vital part of their history. The Russian case is a welcome exception. Among the long lists of materials bought, kept, and used by the Apothecary Chancery, we can find a notable number of American products. The Apothecary Chancery shows us the end use of drugs, completing the story of the early modern global drugs trade from acquisition to prescription.

That completion of the story is possible by accepting the focus of the Russian records on *materia medica*. To do so, we need to think about *materia medica* as material culture. The material culture approach has been increasingly popular in the history of science and medicine. In their edited volume *Ways of Making and Knowing: The Material Culture of Empirical Knowledge* Pamela Smith, Amy Meyers, and Harold J. Cook have argued that materials were often vital to early modern scientific and medical practices, and so "the history of science is not a history of concepts, or at least not that alone, but a history of the making and using of objects to understand the world."[9] Although the precise materials of early modern Russian pharmacy were consumed or lost long ago, the documents that remain are documents about objects.

Indeed, material culture studies has long included a strand of examining objects through texts about those objects. One example is Marianne De Laet and Annemarie Mol's work on the Zimbabwe Bush Pump, in which they substantially rely upon an instruction manual on how to install this object, even as the object itself is available to them.[10] Another is Craig Clunas's *Superfluous Things*, which looks at both Ming-era luxury objects, and the texts, ideas, and words about those objects.[11] This branch of material culture studies is particularly appropriate to the study of lost objects like early modern *materia medica,* and has already been applied by scholars such as Carla Nappi in her work on early modern uses of ginseng.[12] In such cases, we use texts to retrieve something of the objects they are about, thus taking a fundamentally different approach to studies using texts to explore the history of ideas or of historical figures. Through the voluminous records of the Apothecary Chancery on medical drugs we are able to write a material history of objects otherwise lost to us.

Here I particularly follow Pratik Chakrabarti's work on *materia medica.* In *Materials and Medicine,* Chakrabarti shows how European medicine was fundamentally shaped by eighteenth-century European encounters with non-Western knowledge of medicinal materials, in particular those encounters created as a result of British colonialism.[13] My story is no less one of colonialism: The Apothecary Chancery exploited the conquered territories of Russian expansion as well as benefiting from materials they could buy because of Western European conquests in Asia and the Americas. Yet it is also a different story. Chakrabarti showed us the internal workings of materials within one empire; early modern Russian medicine made substantial use of the colonial products of other empires for their *materia medica.*

This focus on materials that were moved through long-distance trade and colonial links raises issues of how to understand objects as they moved through different contexts. The material culture approach again provides models here. Anne Gerritsen and Giorgio Riello deliberately use a plural in the title of their *The Global Lives of Things* to highlight the "transformation of objects through processes of customisation, alteration, and re-combination." Each single object had multiple lives, in the sense of multiple uses and meanings in the different contexts through which it was moved.[14] The use and significance of, say, nutmeg, was different in the various Afro-Eurasian healing traditions that valued it. In following objects, then, we also follow knowledge. This aspect has been highlighted by Pamela Smith in her edited volume *Entangled Itineraries,* which focuses on "entangled itineraries of knowledge-making about specific materials and practices."[15] When we think of nutmeg, we need to think not only of the object, but also of the different ideas about that object at different times and places. In order to understand the general implications of the presence of diverse *materia medica* in early modern Russian records, we must keep in mind not only the origins of the materials, but the context in which they landed. We must remember that these were global objects in Muscovite hands.

DOCTORING TRADITIONS AND THE RUSSIAN EMPIRE

The specificity of the Russian Imperial context is vital here. Writing of the global histories of science, Projit Bihari Mukharji has stated, "The majority of studies look at how non-Western knowledge is transformed into globalized intelligence useful to the 'West.' They do not seek to explore how 'Western' scientific intelligence might have conversely fitted into other, non-Western traditions of natural knowledge."[16] The Russian context allows us to both meet Mukharji's implicit challenge to write histories examining how Western science and medicine was integrated into other knowledge systems, and to complicate it. After all, Russia has a tricky relationship to "the West." Eighteenth-century St Petersburg is commonly presented as Western; seventeenth-century Moscow is not. Yet pre-1700 Russia was integrated with European diplomatic and trading networks, and the major religion was a branch of European Christianity. Moving Samuel Collins's knowledge from Latin into Russian was not entirely a West–East exchange in the way it is usually meant. Yet it was still a blending, or as Mukharji would have it, a braiding, of Western European knowledge into a local non-Western European knowledge system.

The issue of Western versus non-Western, and more broadly local versus foreign, knowledge systems is then also more knotty than the terminological shorthands we commonly use can express. As we have said, Muscovy was not Western Europe, but it was not as different from Western Europe as, say, the Aztec Empire. But in the case of medicine, there were always overlaps. Europeans appropriated the medicines of the Americas because, different as European and Indigenous American societies were, they nevertheless shared certain ideas, notably the utility of plants in medicine. All societies are different, but fundamentally they are also all human groups that grapple with illness and death. The case of Muscovy is significant because it shows how apparent closeness can conceal major fractures. As we will see, ideas that were accepted in Western Europe were taboo in Muscovy; their shared European Christianity did not build a straightforward bridge between their cultures. In that sense, we can then see Muscovy as non-Western, as it was divided from the

West by fundamental chasms regarding bodies and what bodies should consume. What exactly were these Russian concepts? What does the Russian context tell us about *how* to examine Western knowledge blended into non-Western systems of knowledge? And what does it tell us about *why* those blendings happened?

To do this, the first thing we should remember is that the early modern Russian Empire was a sprawling and diverse polity. By 1500, Moscow already dominated the Western Steppe; across the next two and a half centuries, it would swallow up much of the other successor states to the Mongol Empire, expanding south and east to conquer Siberia and eventually territories as far-flung as the Pacific Coast of North America. That empire contained within its massive scope a number of different doctoring traditions, to use another of Mukharji's phrases.[17] Eve Levin has written about Russian folk healers and their use of herbal medicine.[18] Islamic medicine within the pre-1700 Russian Empire is a virtually unexplored topic, but the medical practices of the Muslim populations of the empire like the Tatars may have been similar to that contained in a text by Subḥān Qulī Khan, one of the Khans of Bukhara in the Central Asian Khanate of Bukhara, a fellow Turkic-speaking Muslim.[19] In the early eighteenth century a group of around 150 Tibetan monks travelled to Buryatiia – a region of the Russian Empire near the present-day border with Mongolia – led by the *amchi* Chökyi Ngawang Phüntsog, who became one of the main founders of Tibetan medicine in Buryatiia.[20] Yet before 1700, these diverse traditions were overshadowed by one institution: the Apothecary Chancery, the Russian Imperial medical institution par excellence. The Apothecary Chancery set the rules of legal medical practice within the empire, and has left us the bulk of medical documents from this period, including on unofficial practices, so it is to the Apothecary Chancery that we turn.

By the time Samuel Collins was writing about the global objects of medicine in 1664, he was writing in a very specific Russian Imperial institutional context, one which had been developing across the late sixteenth and early seventeenth centuries. Here, I am using the terms "Russian Empire" and "Russian Imperial" as terms of analysis. Russia itself only formally began to use the term "Imperiia" in the early eighteenth century under Peter the Great. What I call the Russian Empire – the polity centred on Moscow from the 1550s on – is not what Russians of that period called it. Yet "Empire" is not only an issue of contemporary terminology, it is an analytical category. Empires are polities that conquer new territories, link them bureaucratically to the metropole, and use those new territories for settlements or resources. Russia from the conquest of Kazan in 1552, which brought that khanate under their control, until the Treaty of Nerchinsk with the Qing in 1689, which delineated Russia's territorial acquisitions in Asia, certainly fits this model. Indeed, seventeenth-century Russia arguably fits such a definition better than eighteenth-century Russia does, as the latter primarily consolidated and reorganized the territorial gains of the previous century and a half. More importantly, for a work in which colonial materials are key, we need to think in terms of empires. In sum, I use the term "Russian Empire" to describe sixteenth- and seventeenth-century Russia because I believe it is a better definition of the polity with which we are dealing with than simply calling it "Russia."

Within this pre-Petrine Russian Empire, Collins worked for the Apothecary Chancery in which foreign medical practitioners played a major part. Men like Collins were not the only medical practitioners in Muscovy. Like many places in the early modern global world, the East Slavic lands, and indeed the territories that the Russian Empire was colonizing in the early modern period, had multiple practitioners following their own doctoring traditions, between whom and the imported experts of men like Collins there was a fragile peace. The British Indian context has proven especially fruitful for understanding how traditions have coexisted, with Kapil Raj describing knowledge texts produced in that context as "co-constructed" between multiple actors across two continents, and Mukharji's phrase "braided sciences" as a way to understand how different traditions wound around each other. As Mukharji explains, thinking of this as "braiding" helps us understand how traditions consist of different strands that can wind tightly together or unwind from each other, as well as winding or unwinding to one or more strands of other traditions.[21] Mukharji's concept in particular helps us understand the complex coexistences of the doctoring traditions of Muscovy, and how they interacted with doctoring traditions from outside the empire, and with other Imperial Russian practices like diplomacy, religion, and colonization.

The earliest we can clearly identify a bureaucratic institution of official medicine in Russia is the 1570s. The creation of that medical department reified existing divisions between the multiple groups who already coexisted and competed in early modern Russia. Eastern Orthodox Christianity had been the major religion in the East Slavic lands since the

Christianization of Kievan Rus' in the 980s; Muscovy continued this tradition, and the role of Russian Orthodox Christian churchmen as providers of medical treatments. Alongside the churchmen, there were a range of local heterodox healers, whose activities are primarily known from accusations against them, and who were commonly portrayed as practising a combination of herbal medicine, heterodox prayers, magic, and divination. And then there were the predecessors to Samuel Collins, foreign physicians, surgeons and apothecaries, primarily from Western Europe, whose personal positions at court would eventually be transformed into a part of bureaucratic medicine.

Religious healing by officially recognized Russian Orthodox Christian churchmen was a major part of healing in Muscovy, even as it was not directly a part of the Apothecary Chancery. Rather, these two branches of licit healing coexisted fairly peacefully, with the department sending supplies, and occasionally even patients to the churchmen.[22] Often the church took in the soul-sick [*dushevnaia bolezn'*], something akin to what we would now call mental illness, although people with certain physical illnesses, in particular the falling sickness [*paduchaia bolezn'*], a term often conflated with epilepsy, sometimes also turned to religious healing. This religious healing involved particular spaces, like saints' shrines at which the sick prayed for recovery, particular objects like relics, and noted individuals. Both Avakuum Petrov and Archbishop Afanasii of Kholmogory, major figures on opposite sides of the religious Schism of the 1660s, were famous for their medical practices.[23] Significantly, their healing also differed: Afanasii of Kholmogory wrote a pharmacy text on the creation and usage of medical drugs; Petrov believed true healing came only from confessing sins and reconnecting to God. Russian Orthodox Christian healing traditions were multiple and were braided loosely to each other, and to court medicine.

Magic was never far from medicine in the pre-modern East Slavic lands. The modern Russian term for doctor – *vrach* – is derived from the verb *vrachevati*, which in the sixteenth century could mean either to heal or to ensorcell; the term *balii* could mean either a magical or a medical practitioner; and the word *volkhv*, although most commonly used to mean wizards or non-Christian religious figures, was on occasion also used to refer to medical doctors.[24] Magic at court was a substantial concern to the Muscovites.[25] Herbal healing was also worrisome, for similar reasons. Courtly magic everywhere was about political and dynastic intrigue; court medicine also held possibilities for such shenanigans. Local healers were often in a relationship with elite personages, and so this raised the possibility that they might be convinced or coerced into harming the tsar.[26] Not all such local healers had a bad reputation: one sixteenth-century tale, *Petr and Fevroniia,* presents the fictional folk-healer Fevroniia as better than trained medical practitioners, as she succeeds in healing Prince Petr's illness where they had failed.[27] In the overwhelming majority of cases, information about these unofficial healers comes from documents written by their detractors, and so our understanding of their practices, motivations, and actions will always be coloured by that. We can at least say that there was a group of local practitioners who offered a range of services to understand and manipulate nature, and healing human bodies was commonly within their range of services.

Herbal medical drugs were a part of their practice. The *Domostroi,* a household advice text that may have been partly taken from a Western European work and which circulated Muscovy in multiple manuscripts from the mid-sixteenth century on, condemns healers as sorcerers and forbids the reader from consulting such practitioners, or indeed having any dealings whatsoever with them.[28] Similarly, the mid-sixteenth-century Russian Orthodox Church text the *Stoglav* condemns *zelinichestvo,* an abstract noun derived from the Slavonic word for herb and meaning treatment with herbs, or perhaps more generally knowledge of herbs.[29] It is not entirely clear what the *Stoglav* is condemning: herbs were used for a range of purposes, and in the sixteenth century were associated with both poisoning and witchcraft.[30] Again, the views contained in the *Stoglav* come from the persecutors of those practitioners, not the practitioners themselves. But it is interesting that they were in part condemned for prescribing consumable medical drugs. Heterodox practices appear to us braided together with official views on such practices, because that is how we access that world.

By the time the *Stoglav* was compiled in 1550, the courtly elite of Russia had an alternative both to the licit practice of churchmen and to the illicit practices of the heterodox practitioners: invited foreign medical practitioners. In 1472, the Byzantine Princess Sofia Palaeologa travelled to Moscow to marry Grand Prince Ivan III; a physician was a part of her retinue. Late fifteenth- and early sixteenth-century court documents and chronicles make scattered references to a handful of such medical practitioners. In 1490, Ivan III asked the Holy Roman Emperor for a physician; in the same year, Vienna sent him one Leon Zhidovin. In the 1510s, doctor Teofil worked for the court, recruited from Prussia, as did Marko Grek a subject of the Ottoman Sultan (not to be confused with the churchman Maxim Grek, also active in Russia in the same period).[31] By the early sixteenth century the Moscow court employed perhaps one or two such foreign medical practitioners at a time, whose medical practices were bound tightly together with diplomatic and dynastic practices.

There were specific reasons to recruit foreign medical practitioners. Eve Levin has argued that foreign servitors, dependent upon the tsar for their position, were seen as less susceptible to bribes to harm the tsar than local practitioners, already indebted to other lords, may have been.[32] As will so often be the case with our story, here we see only hints of this medical world, but the hints are fairly consistent: heterodox healers available to the elite and commoners alike; religious healers focused on Christian-centred diseases and cures; and a court moving towards foreign servitors for security reasons. Doctoring traditions in Muscovy were always braided together with social and political concerns.

These practitioners were commonly recruited through the westward-facing diplomacy of the late fifteenth and sixteenth centuries, as Muscovy turned away from the fading remnants of the Golden Horde in the east and instead looked west to Europe. Indeed, this trend of recruiting medical practitioners from Western Europe continued into the seventeenth and eighteenth centuries, despite Moscow's having diplomatic links to other Eurasian courts and being aware of other doctoring traditions. Islamic medicine, for example, was never practised at the Moscow court. One reason for this was antagonism towards Islam. The level of animosity of the Russian elite towards Muslims waxed and waned, but we do see evidence of suspicion of Muslims in this period. In 1617 the Shah of Iran sent Christian holy relics to Moscow in an attempt to head off a brewing conflict; these relics were initially regarded with suspicion.[33] An Apothecary Chancery document uses language common to anti-Islamic diatribes to discuss coffee, a beverage associated with Muslim lands.[34] Such suspicion of Islam meant Muslim medical practitioners would not have fulfilled the security requirements Levin has highlighted.

Moreover, there were other places from which to source medical practitioners, particularly regions with which the Russian court had more harmonious relations than with the Muslim lands. Maria Unkovskaya and

Sabine Dumschat have demonstrated that the practitioners of the Apothecary Chancery overwhelmingly came from specific Western European regions, notably the Protestant countries England, the Netherlands, and certain of the German Lands; before the middle of the seventeenth century, the Apothecary Chancery employed no Russian as a medical practitioner.[35] No extant document explicitly explains this trend. However, we can situate the medical situation within other contexts. Even with the existence of contacts elsewhere, the Moscow court was increasingly interested in this period in the cultural practices, material goods, and practical expertise of Western Europe. We can see this in the general scheme of foreign experts in early modern Russia, who were overwhelmingly from Western Europe.[36] The preferences of Muscovite diplomacy and elite society shaped the personnel of official medicine.

For the early part of the sixteenth century, what we have is names of practitioners; it is only in the 1570s, during the reign of Tsar Ivan IV (also known as The Terrible), that we see mentions of a bureaucratic institution. In 1572, a century after Sophia Palaeologa's arrival with her personal physician, an inventory of the royal household noted the presence of several texts belonging to the Apothecary Building, *Aptechnaia izba*.[37] That first mention of the Apothecary Building, as a marginal note in a document substantially concerned with other matters, is typical for the documentary traces of that institution. The only documents that can be definitively traced as being the product of that department are eight prescriptions from the early 1580s.[38] Otherwise, the department appears only on the edges of other affairs, making the evaluation of its activities and purposes particularly tricky. One point is noteworthy. The earlier practitioners – Bülow, Teofil, and others – were not associated with a department; rather, they seem to have been individual members of court. The Apothecary Building was a department within the bureaucracy, unwinding imported foreign doctoring from its earlier association with individuals and braiding it more tightly with the bureaucracy.

Significantly, the Apothecary Building also seems to have been a department based in a separate physical structure. This may well relate to its name: of all the possible contemporary medical-related terms that could have been used here – *lechebnyi, vrachebnyi, lekarskii, tselitel'nii* – the department makes reference to apothecary work in particular. Medical affairs may have been formalized into a housed department to ease

Table 1
Origins of Foreign Medical Practitioners in the Apothecary Chancery, 1600–1696

Period	*Origin unknown*	*German Lands*	*Ruthenia, Poland, Lithuania*	*England and Scotland*	*The Low Countries*	*Other European**	*Total*
1600–1620	6	4	1	2	3	1	17
1620–1640	15	2	0	7	6	5	35
1640–1660	13	8	17	5	4	4	51
1660–1680	13	25	21	6	5	13	83
1680–1696	31	37	11	3	5	14	101

Adapted from Dumschat, *Ausländischer Mediziner*, 105.

* Denmark, Greece, Sweden, Italy, France

the creation of medical drugs. The arrival of British apothecary James Frencham in 1581 is often taken as a key stage in the formalization of official Russian medicine, and his arrival could mark the importation of equipment to stock the Apothecary Building.[39] Most importantly, once again we return to the central idea of this book: for early modern Russia, medicine meant medical drugs.

References to an official medical department die away in the 1590s, to reappear in the 1610s and 1620s as Russia emerged from the dynastic crisis of the Time of Troubles with the new Romanov dynasty in place.[40] From the 1620s, the Moscow court's medical department is known as the *Aptekarskii prikaz,* the Apothecary Chancery. Its exact relationship to the earlier Apothecary Building is unclear, in part because we know so little about the earlier institution.[41] We do know that there were similarities between the two institutions. Both were run by a Russian noble, usually a close relative of the Tsaritsa, had a building in or near the Kremlin complex, were staffed by Moscow clerks and foreign medical practitioners, and exchanged documents with the other parts of early modern Russia's imperial bureaucracy.[42] There may have been a difference in patient circle: we know both institutions treated court figures, but the Apothecary Chancery also treated the army from at least the 1630s. The Apothecary Chancery would remain in business until the early eighteenth century and was the major official institution of early modern Russian medicine, also providing us with the overwhelming majority of extant materials on early modern Russian medicine.[43]

The Apothecary Chancery was initially based within the Moscow Kremlin, and later moved to a building just outside the Kremlin complex. By the middle of the seventeenth century, the department had more than one apothecary garden in Moscow.[44] It also had several outposts, such as a storehouse in Rzhev, and regional centres in Novgorod in the north and Kiev in the south, and made unsuccessful attempts to set up further regional branches in Vologda in the north, and Kazan in the east.[45] The Apothecary Chancery was a part of the *prikaznaia sistema*, commonly referred to as the chancery system, an Imperial Russian bureaucracy that consisted of multiple linked departments. Departments were created and closed down across the century, with around seventy in operation at any one time, covering military affairs of various kinds, dealing with foreign connections, tracking service lands, collecting taxes, and administering newly conquered territories. The Apothecary Chancery was integrated into this system through exchange of documents: it asked regional officials to collect plants for medicines, received requests from military departments to examine wounded soldiers, and was ordered to provide expert testimony in trials.[46] Across the seventeenth century, the imported doctoring traditions from Western Europe were more and more closely braided with imperial practices.

By the 1620s, the Apothecary Chancery was established and functioning; in the second half of the seventeenth century it was substantially rearranged. In 1654, the Apothecary Chancery changed its previous strategy of recruiting medical practitioners from Western Europe to training Russians as both apothecaries and field surgeons.[47] Both relate to the issue of military medicine. The Apothecary Chancery had been providing surgeons and medicines to the Russian army from at least the 1630s, so the expanded staff allowed the department not only to send out surgeons to more regiments, but also to create the increasingly large quantities of medicines required by an institution that supplied the large (and growing) court and the army. The mid-century date of these changes makes sense. Tsar Aleksei Mikhailovich was more of a reformer than his father Mikhail Fedorovich.[48] The year 1654 saw the start of the Russo-Polish war, as well as an outbreak of plague in many parts of central Russia, both of which issues would be better resolved with a more robust medical department.

In 1673, the Apothecary Chancery was again reformed, this time being split into two branches. The newly created New Pharmacy [*Novaia apte-*

ka] dealt with ordinary Muscovites, providing them with officially approved medicine. The rest of the Apothecary Chancery, now called the Old Pharmacy [*Staraia apteka*] or Upper Pharmacy [*Verkhniaia apteka*], dealt with the needs of the court, treating high-ranking patients and providing advice, and also the needs of the army, sending them medicines and medics. Such an occurrence was entirely normal for chancery development: the larger a chancery became and the more numerous its duties, the more complex its internal structure.[49] The Apothecary Chancery continued to operate in this new, bicameral iteration until the end of the seventeenth century. By the late seventeenth century, the doctoring traditions of the Apothecary Chancery were itself beginning to unravel into separate strands.

As the Apothecary Chancery became more involved in prescribing to ordinary Muscovites like soldiers, it was also drawn into investigating and prosecuting medical malpractice in the city. The high tide of such concerns came in 1701. In this year, Tsar Peter I, better known as Peter the Great, enacted legislation that would both shut down market stalls selling medical drugs, and establish Moscow-based licensed apothecaries.[50] These men were the first private individuals to be granted official permission to practise medicine (although Apothecary Chancery medical practitioners had some rights to maintain a private practice); once again, priority was given to the making of drugs over all other kinds of medical practice.

Although the Apothecary Chancery was so central to the pharmacy reform of 1701, the department did not long survive that period as it was slowly pulled apart across the first two decades of the eighteenth century. This heralded not only the end of the Apothecary Chancery itself but also of the monopolistic approach to official medicine it had represented. Although the Medical Chancellery [*Meditsinskaia kantseliariia*], the short-lived successor to the Apothecary Chancery, still provided some services for the military in the early eighteenth century, increasingly the armed forces preferred to have their own medical services. The Military Statute of 1716 increased the scope of the army's already-existing medical wing; the 1720 Naval Statute did the same for the navy.[51] This was not a destruction of the Apothecary Chancery, as its concerns, possessions, and staff would shape eighteenth-century Russian science and medicine. Rather, this was a shattering of the department, and a dispersal of its valuable parts to new institutional homes.

The end of the Apothecary Chancery was formalized in 1721 when a Senate decree put all its remaining employees, buildings, and materials under the control of the newly created Medical Chancellery.[52] That department itself was not long for the world, as it would be replaced by the Medical College in 1763; its documentary trace leaves an even lighter footprint, as its records are preserved only from 1737 on.[53] Its replacement, the Medical College, was a rather different animal, the product of the reforms of that other famous eighteenth-century Russian ruler, Catherine II (popularly known as Catherine the Great). There was also a geographical shift: the hub of seventeenth-century official Russian medicine was always the Moscow Kremlin complex; after the establishment of St Petersburg in 1703 the Medical Chancellery worked in both places, with institutions in both the old and the new capital. These changes concealed deeper continuities: many of the Medical Chancellery's staff had worked, or were the children of men who had worked, in the Apothecary Chancery. By the eighteenth century, the imported Western European doctoring tradition had both unwound from its early association with diplomacy and internally unwound, to become multiple threads all increasingly tightly wound together with the business of the Russian empire.

THE QUESTION OF GLOBALIZATION

As early modern Russian medicine relied heavily on long-distance trading links to supply the ingredients for medical drugs, including on the newly created transatlantic routes, we need to think about globalization. The idea of a pre-modern global world, of early modern globalization, and when and why those concepts might be useful, is fraught. Some scholars have argued that medieval Afro-Eurasia or the early modern Atlantic world can fruitfully be analyzed as being global, but others feel "global" can productively and meaningfully be applied only to more recent historical periods. There are some early modernists who feel that early modern globalization is a vital concept to the field, and others who think it should be dismissed. Those who do agree that early modern globalization is a useful concept do not always agree on what it was, and when it happened. Considering American products in early modern Moscow inevitably requires making an intervention into such scholarly debates.

An important point in my conception of Muscovy's global moment is specificity. Global connections – meaning long-distance links – and globalization – meaning how and when those links evolved – are capacious concepts. To discuss the global, we could talk about commodities, trade, value, and prices, or we could discuss communications and knowledge exchange, or travel and migration. Looking at commodities in the early modern period, then, involves considering one kind of global, not constructing an overall concept of what "global" is. Even more specifically, here we are dealing with medical commodities, rather than bulk items or luxury goods, and focusing on indirect trade, as those commodities were commonly coming from regions with which the Russian Empire did not have a direct connection. We then get a model of how to think about such situations, which were not uncommon in the early modern world, and also how to build other specific models of limited, regional experiences of the global. This then leads to the question, what can considering Muscovy's *materia medica* tell us about the controversial issue of early modern globalization?

The idea that the pre-modern world could be thought of as global dates back to world systems theory and works like Janet Abu-Lughod's *Before European Hegemony: The World System AD 1250–1350*.[54] More recently, a number of scholars have argued for a specific value to thinking of the pre-modern world as global, such as Monica Green, who has contended that pre-modern pandemics like the Black Death are better understood as global phenomena.[55] Particularly useful for our purposes here is Geraldine Heng's work. Heng argues that we should see the interconnectivities of the world as "globalities," a set of long-distance connections specific to a period. She further argues for an "asynchrony of global temporalities," meaning that different long-distance connections formed or dissolved at different times.[56] Both ideas provide a roadmap for thinking of Moscow as one node in a global world, and how Moscow's experience of that world was specific to Moscow, even as it reveals broader trends.

Other historians criticize the idea of a pre-modern global, and even the idea of global history at all. In 2017, Jeremy Adelman proclaimed global history to be dead. Adelman claimed global history to be a product of a now-past era of international co-operation and too focused on the idea of integration and interdependence, to the neglect of equally important narratives of separation and disintegration.[57] Adelman's article, rather than prompting despair in the global history community, instead provoked defences. Richard Drayton and David Motadel have argued that although the specific context from which global history has emerged might be dead, global history cannot be. They point to other historiographical moments, noting how scholars who do not directly practise, for example, history from below, nevertheless have to take account of the peoples and processes such approaches highlighted.[58] The bell cannot be unrung. Having seen the ways in which history has been shaped by global processes, we must continue to take account of those processes, even as we acknowledge the problems in doing so.

There are other responses one can make to Adelman's concerns. It is important to note that global histories do not have to be histories only of integration and interdependence; the recent edited volume by Erica Charters, Marie Houllemare, and Peter H. Wilson on early modern violence in global context is one example of a different kind of global history.[59] Alternatively, we can take the example of sassafras. Sassafras, a tree that grows along the eastern seaboard of North America, was initially part of the medical practices of several Native American nations, including the Timucua of present-day Florida. Across the sixteenth and seventeenth centuries, European invaders appropriated the Timucuan knowledge of sassafras, acquired sassafras examples, and sold them across Afro-Eurasia. At the same time, Europeans murdered the Timucua through a combination of active combat and violent disregard for the impact of virgin soil epidemics.[60] Processes that were constructive, in the sense of making new connections, practices, or things, were also often destructive. The early modern period was the violent remaking of the world.

Global history is a fraught concept; early modern globalization may be even more so. A number of scholars have looked at the major changes to long-distance trade and travel during the long sixteenth century as evidence of early modern globalization. The most specific claim is that of Dennis Flynn and Arturo Giraldez, who take the founding of Manila in 1571, which facilitated the ability to trade circuitously around the globe, as the start of globalization.[61] More generally, the term is used by scholars to refer to the period from the late fifteenth to the early eighteenth centuries as one in which major changes were made to long-distance connections, and during which objects and knowledge circulated the world in different ways than they had before.[62] Given the prominence of new American drugs in Eurasia to studies of the early modern drugs trade, early modern globalization has been a fundamental concept for such studies.[63] The concept of globalization is unavoidable when considering the drugs trade.

This does not mean it is universally accepted. Even historians who find the concept of pre-modern global useful have criticized the idea of applying the term "globalization" to early periods. Heng rejects its application to the pre-modern world, concerned that doing so erases the specificities of our current global moment.[64] Jan de Vries has criticized the idea of an early modern globalization by citing economic history concerns over the extent and measurability of change.[65] Looking at African history, Frederick Cooper expresses concerns similar to Adelman's that thinking globally glosses over breakdowns in favour of writing of successes and connections, as well as ignoring local stories.[66] De Vries argues that the concept of globalization is too big for the early modern period; Cooper argues that it is too big for any period.

So then why do I insist upon framing this study not only as global history, but a history of globalization? The criticisms of both can be essentialized to this: there has been a mismatch between the ideas of global and globalization and the material being studied, leading to those approaches concealing or misrepresenting more than they reveal. It is my contention that the concepts of the global and globalization are appropriate to use in the context of early modern Russian *materia medica* because they reveal important aspects we would otherwise struggle to explain. In contrast to Cooper's concerns as an Africanist that the concept of globalization hurts or hides his subject, as a Russianist I find that the same concept – used cautiously – has huge potential to reveal vital aspects of Russian history that we cannot otherwise consider.

I then use the terms "global" and "globalization" in specific ways for specific reasons. When I say "global," I am talking about a network of long-distance trade and exchange, or the objects that could only be obtained through said network. In the sixteenth century, Muscovy's *materia medica* were already global. By this I mean they were being obtained through a Hengian kind of specific Muscovite globality of a particular combination of long-distance connections across Afro-Eurasia that was similar to the connections of other major cities but also fundamentally unique to Moscow.[67] It is possible to understand the particular combinations of ingredients that went into a single drug that we will see in the 1580s only by thinking about those objects as global.

When I say "globalization," I am talking about a limited globalization, the shift in Moscow's global links that fundamentally changed Russian *materia medica*. In the seventeenth century, the specific Muscovite globality of the previous century shifted substantially with the entrance of American drugs as a major new focus, linking Moscow to the Atlantic world. Muscovy's entrance into the Atlantic world was temporally disjointed from that of, say, Spain. This was a key point of Moscow's "asynchrony of global temporalities," as Moscow and the Russian Empire more generally joined this post-contact world after Spain and the Native American nations of the eastern seaboard.[68] We could talk of this in Hengian terms of a shifting globality from the sixteenth to the seventeenth century.[69] But I chose to use the more popular and widespread term of globalization, simply because it is more familiar. Muscovy's *materia medica* was dependent on global links, which went through a major global shift during the seventeenth century that had long-term consequences. We can reasonably call this globalization and use that phrase to highlight an important fact about this history.

Embracing the complications of calling this a story of globalization also allows us to bring in literature on both global science and the global drugs trade that enrich how we understand the Russian situation. As Fati Fan noted in 2012, there has been a global turn in the history of science, in part occasioned by the need to deal with the long-term global movement of objects that has shaped scientific ideas and practices.[70] Early modernists have played a significant role in this historiographical moment, from Kapil Raj's now-classic *Relocating Modern Science* to more recent edited volumes by Jorge Cañizares-Esguerra and Helge Wendt.[71] As Cañizares-Esguerra has put it, "Scholars are just now beginning to realize that the European Renaissance and Enlightenment were not European inventions but vast encyclopaedias of hybrid global knowledge processed and packaged in Europe."[72] Focusing on Moscow, a site connected to Western Europe but never entirely part of Latinate Western European natural historical knowledge circles, permits us a new perspective on this knowledge.

Thinking about globalization also helps us think about the early modern drugs trade as global, and conceptualizations that see the link between the drugs trade and early modern global processes as fundamental. Brett Neilson and Mohammed Bamyeh have argued that drugs are a material manifestation of global processes, and that we have to think about global mobilities if we think about drugs.[73] Building on this, Benjamin Breen has asked, "[a]re drugs, then, not modern, but distinctively early modern, in the sense that both the term itself and its societal role emerged in tandem with the rise of colonial exploitation, state formation, and global trade in the three centuries after Columbus?"[74] For Breen, drugs, global trade, and early modernity are inextricably linked. We have many works on the specifics of the movement of drugs through this early modern global world which Breen sees as so essentially entangled. Looking to Moscow we can see the effects of this global world when it came to rest.

MUSCOVITE GLOBAL SCIENCE

Thus far we have spoken of this *materia medica* project as if its Russianness were merely a happenstance, as if this were a case study almost accidentally focused on Russia, but which primarily tells us things external to Russia. And this book can be read in such a way. A reader uninterested in Russian history per se and concerned only with the problem of early modern globalization, of material culture and the history of science and medicine, or the early modern drugs trade, could work their way through this work thinking only of those issues. But this book is also about early modern Russia.

For those of us who are interested in Russia qua Russia, looking at medical drugs gives us a vital and underconsidered view on our region. We are here in part concerned with knowledge, knowledge about what drugs were and how to use them. Knowledge is bounded and shaped by many things, such as the other identities of the knowledge creators, their place in society, and the support of or opposition to certain kinds of knowledge. A clichéd and apparently immortal issue for science is its relationship to religion, which has rarely been as antithetical as some would argue but has always been significant. Society has shaped knowledge, but knowledge has also shaped society; the two are ever locked into a complex symbiosis. As Russianists, the question for us then is what does this case study tell us about the specificities of knowledge in Muscovy? And how did those specificities interact with Muscovite society and culture more broadly?

A major issue here is continuities and discontinuities. This project covers the period 1534 to 1750, crossing two significant boundaries of historiography. This book begins by traversing the border between the sixteenth and seventeenth centuries, a crossing made many times by social, political, and cultural histories, but less common in histories of

Russian science and medicine. One strand of scholarship concerns medieval Russian science, with Rem Aleksandrovich Morozov in particular working on multiple pre-modern, and typically pre-1600, Slavonic medical and astrological manuscripts; significant work has also been done comparing the 1534 and 1616 Slavonic *Garden of Health* manuscripts.[75] In contrast, studies of official medicine typically take the 1620s, the beginning of good Apothecary Chancery record preservation, as the starting point.[76] Yet these groups of sources have a major similarity: the pre-1620s herbals are as concerned with medical drugs as was the Apothecary Chancery. Studying *materia medica*, then, both allows and requires us to skip across the narrow yet significant temporal boundary from the 1616 *Garden of Health* to the 1620s Apothecary Chancery files.

At the other chronological end of this project, we also cross into the eighteenth century. The reign of Peter the Great was long considered the defining line between Muscovy and "Imperial Russia" for cultural, political, and social histories; the establishment of the Academy of Sciences in 1725 typically played the same role for histories of Russian science. That Rubicon of the early eighteenth century has been crossed several times now, but rarely by historians of science and medicine. Those of us writing on the Apothecary Chancery typically end our studies as the department's records peter out in the 1690s–1710s.[77] There are then works such as Loren Graham's classic study of Russian science that begins after 1700, and that of Andreas Renner, which looks at Russian medicine of the mid- to late eighteenth century.[78] Those of us who focus on the seventeenth century rarely venture into the eighteenth, and vice versa. Yet here, again, the material demands that this boundary be traversed. The *Garden of Health*, the Apothecary Chancery files, and Medical Chancellery, all shared a mutual affinity with *materia medica*. Following *materia medica* builds us a long and complex road two hundred years long.

The issue of Muscovy's interest in *materia medica* also takes us to the issue of early modern Russia's international links. We have long left behind the idea that Muscovy was cut off from the rest of the early modern world, with a number of scholars highlighting Russia's connections to Western Europe, Asia, and Middle Eastern polities like the Ottoman Empire.[79] This book builds on that work, as it considers how *materia medica* flowed through those same connections. It also reveals a rather different geography. At least by the 1580s, Russia was using materials from Africa, a region that appears rarely in histories of early modern Russia.[80] Russia's links with the Americas similarly are all but absent in this period, being written almost exclusively through the history of the short-lived Russian colonies in Pacific North America, which are typically framed as beginning with a voyage across the Bering Sea in 1732.[81] Yet the presence of American *materia medica* in Russia predates that voyage by more than a century, as well as shifting the focus from the Pacific to the Atlantic world. To write about *materia medica* in Muscovy is to redraw the map of early modern Russia's international interactions.

Focusing on the Apothecary Chancery's expertise on *materia medica* also requires us to think about what how we define science and expertise. The work of the Western European physicians easily fits into standard definitions; the activities of the herb collectors also fits within currently accepted ideas of artisan expertise.[82] Yet both groups were a part of a broader world of Slavic views on nature. As I and others discussed in a special edition of *ВИВЛІОѲИКА* devoted to this theme in 2018, over the past decade and a half there has been a "natural turn" in early modern Russian studies.[83] That turn focuses on how Muscovites viewed the powers and possibilities of the natural world, and includes work by Valerie Kivelson on cartography, by Kivelson, Eve Levin, E.B. Smilianskaia, and A.S. Lavrov on witchcraft, and by A.B. Ippolitova on ethno-botanical works.[84] Once the remit of the Apothecary Chancery began expanding in the late seventeenth century, the department would directly interact with such views as it provided expert testimony in witchcraft trials. The Apothecary Chancery was a hybrid institution, sitting at the nexus of medieval Slavonic science, popular Muscovite views on nature, Russian bureaucratic principles, Western European expertise, and global *materia medica*, to create a Muscovite global science.

* * *

The centre of Muscovy's medical world was always medical drugs. This concern emerged from an earlier conflation of potion, poison, and drug into the phrase *zel'ia*, and entered the Apothecary Chancery language via that department's reliance upon earlier Muscovite oaths of service and fealty. Those concerns were significant. Not only did the department have their servitors pledge to create only good drugs, it also punished them for infractions. That drive to root out bad medical drugs led to a mission creep, first of the department being involved in investigating individual cases of medical malpractice and healing-related witchcraft, then by the late seventeenth-century broader police actions against Moscow-based unofficial medical drug peddlers as a group. Chapter 1 establishes how the centrality of medical drugs to Russian understandings of medicine shaped both official and unofficial practices.

Chapter 2 looks at which natural objects were considered appropriate to put in good medicines. The overwhelming majority of medical drug ingredients in Russia from the sixteenth to the eighteenth century were plants. Moreover, that focus on botanicals led early modern official Russian medicine to use global substances. In the sixteenth century, the court was already reading about and using ingredients from North Africa, East Asia, and Southeast Asia, as well as local herbs and Western European products. At the start of the seventeenth century they also began importing American botanicals, the only American products to be in serious use in Russia before the eighteenth century. This enthusiasm for global botanical medicines from both Afro-Eurasia and the Americas continued into the eighteenth century.

While botanical medical ingredients were accepted, chemical medicine was less so. Chapter 3 looks at the turbulent history of chemical medicine in early modern Russia and what it tells us about the decision-making processes of the Apothecary Chancery. Medical practitioners from Western Europe were early promoters of this group of ingredients, but there was notable resistance from Russian officials, even as late as the 1690s. Eventually chemicals would find a place within official Russian medicine, but it took a century and substantial lobbying from the medical practitioners. This shows a co-construction of rules between Western European experts and local officials.

The materials of medicine also clashed with religious proscriptions. Chapter 4 examines the category of flesh-based medicines, focusing particularly on mumia, powdered mummified human flesh, and theriac, a compound medicine including vipers' flesh. Russian and Western European documents both specifically note how these medicaments were unacceptable to the Russian court in the early seventeenth century, a ban fundamentally based on Muscovite Orthodox Christian ideas of the body and rules on consumption. Under Peter the Great, Russian culture changed, and with it the status of these two medicines as well, eventually leading to acceptance of these medicines. Within the Muscovite cosmology of Russian Orthodox Christianity, the materiality and status of the human body was key, and so materials of medicine always had to interact with rules about human bodies that came from society, not just science.

All of these materials we encounter via their documentary traces, a topic addressed in chapter 5, which looks at those textual objects directly. The Apothecary Chancery owned and created numerous texts; indeed, one of its key functions was to create reports using authoritative texts to address specific questions of concern to the court and the bureaucracy of empire, which then fed into trials, legislation, and licensing. In the eighteenth century, some practices of texts and authority changed. There were new institutions, and Russia found a use for mass-produced printed texts. Yet the Apothecary Chancery's successor, the Medical Chancellery, still used the same practices of investigation to produce reports in legal cases which went on to inform new legislation, following the pattern established earlier in the Apothecary Chancery's work. Half-hidden under all these changes, the textual practices of the Apothecary Chancery remained.

* * *

The end of this book is a pharmacy regulation that aimed to control all drug creation, prescription, and consumption across an empire that covered one-eighth of the world's land surface. But to get to such an ambitious gambit, we need to begin with something much less far-reaching: the service oath of one department in the Moscow Kremlin in the 1620s.

1

The Importance of *Lekarstva*

All around the early modern world people tried to maintain health and treat sickness. We can find much in common in these attempts, but we can also find differences both between and within regions, differences scholars have categorized with a range of terms. Projit Bihari Mukharji has, as we have already seen, created the term "doctoring traditions" to discuss the interaction of approaches he sees in the modern South Asian context.[1] In contrast, John Slater, Maríaluz López-Terrada, and José Pardo-Tomás use the phrase "medical cultures" to express something similar about the early modern Spanish Empire. "[M]edicine," they write, "constitutes, on the one hand, a varied form of cultural practice and production, and on the other, a significant matrix for the intersection of a wide range of cultural phenomena (political, literary, religious, or otherwise)."[2] Mukharji, Slater, López-Terrada, and Pardo-Tomás are all concerned with understanding medicine as having different traditions that interact, change, and are changed by both other medical traditions and non-medical ideas and practices. Fundamental to this is the idea that each tradition has something particular about it, a mutable yet coherent core of ideas and practices that constitute the tradition itself. To understand medicine or doctoring in a particular time and place, we need to understand what that core was.

When we examine the official Russian medicine of the sixteenth, seventeenth, and early eighteenth centuries, one central concern jumps out: medical drugs, in Russian *lekarstva* [pl.; *lekarstvo* sing.]. The first complete medical book translated into Slavonic was an herbal. The only extant records from the sixteenth-century official medical department, the *Aptechnaia izba*, are prescriptions. Across the seventeenth and into the eighteenth century the staff of the Apothecary Chancery and the Medical Chancellery swore oaths to create medical drugs well, produced medical drugs, wrote books about medical drugs both for the departments and for their own purposes, and were deeply involved in investigating and legislating against the incorrect creation of medical drugs above all other kinds of medical malpractice. The core of early modern official Russian medicine was drugs.

As the major set of documents for studying early modern Russian medicine comes from the Apothecary Chancery, we can see this core concern both in that department's records and in its intersections with other medical practices within the Russian Empire and other aspects of life in that context. That fixation on medical drugs emerged out of an older fear of malefic magic and poisoning, and a conflation of spell, poison, and medicine in the word *zel'ia*.[3] Anxiety regarding malefic magic and poisoning certainly traces as far back as the fourteenth century and shows up in both official documents like oaths and in the testimony of unofficial healers that we find caught up in witchcraft and malpractice trials. That concern continues even as the Russian language evolved over this period, with the emergence of the modern word for medical drugs, *lekarstvo*. The concept that natural objects had a specific power to help and harm human bodies was both long-lived and widespread in early modern Russia.

The focus on *materia medica* substantially shaped both the practices of official Russian medicine and the interactions of officialdom with unofficial healing. At the start of the seventeenth century, the Apothecary Chancery took pains to regulate the production of medicines above all other medical practices in the department, with pre-emptive rules, investigations, and punishments for infractions. By the latter part of the century, the department was increasingly involved in both witchcraft trials and investigations into medical malpractice by unofficial practitioners, specifically when medical drugs were involved. Those malpractice investigations themselves spiralled, moving from case-by-case affairs to a broader investigation into the market for unofficial medicines itself. The Muscovite concern over consumable medicines fundamentally shaped early modern Russian medicine, determining both official practices and the prosecution of unofficial activities. The central concern of early modern Russian medicine was medical drugs, and so we can begin our examination of that medical culture with the texts that most directly demonstrate that specific issue.

FIRST, DO NO HARM

One prominent place in which we can see the concern over medical drugs is in the Apothecary Chancery's service oaths. When medical practitioners joined the Apothecary Chancery, they agreed to a standard of practice and behaviour as set out in a long oath. In a version from the 1620s we find the following passage:

> I pledge ... not to spoil [patients' health] with any kind of affair nor with any kind of cunning and not to give an evil herb or root ... not to put unclean mumia nor any evil snake poison nor other poisonous animal nor reptile nor bird [nor] any evil and unclean compound that could harm health into medicines ... to watch vigilantly over my colleagues in preparing all concoctions and in all measures which are created for their, the Tsar's, health so that they [my colleagues] do not put into [those] concoctions anything bad nor substitute an evil herb for a good.[4]

The oath does not contain that now quintessential phrase of medical ethics – "primum non nocere" (first, do no harm) – but neither does the text from which the phrase supposedly originates, the Hippocratic oath.[5] The popularity of this phrase seems to stem rather from its concise expression of what is seen as a fundamental principle of medical ethics of all periods, that physicians not use their knowledge for harm. The Apothecary Chancery oath agrees with the spirit of this: a central issue of this passage is that no medicine be prescribed that could *harm health*. This key document marking the start of medical service in the Apothecary Chancery thus emphasized in particular the issue of medical drugs as central to the maintenance or harm of someone's health.

This pledge to avoid harming health by careful attention to medical drugs, then, was the start of medical service at the seventeenth-century Russian court. Yet in all cases the association between court and practitioner pre-dated the oath taking, often by many months. The vast majority of medical practitioners working for the Apothecary Chancery were not Russian but rather recruits from Western Europe. They often received their first paycheque before even arriving in Russia, an honorarium to defray the expenses of travel. That travel, over hundreds of miles and taking weeks if not months, was their first act after having accepted their position, recruited by their monarch, a Russian ambassador, or a merchant in Russian service.[6] Yet the oath remained vital. Every practitioner had to take it, swearing on the Bible appropriate to his creed, before providing the least medical assistance. Violation of the oath was serious business: infractions of its precepts led to corporal punishment or dismissal. The Apothecary Chancery oath is notably detailed, taking up several pages of permitted, required, and banned activities. In this lies its great value to the historical study of medicine in early modern Russia: in this document Muscovites poured out their neuroses, revealed their obsessions, and fixed the limitations of their imagined official medical world. Oaths, in a very real sense, were the limits of that world, and the limits of that world were primarily arranged around medical drugs.

The importance of the focus on medical drugs can also be shown by considering the aspects of contemporary medical practice to which the oath does not devote particular attention. Drugs are powerful, and therefore both useful and dangerous. Such a description could also be applied to bloodletting, the practice of opening a vein to remove excess blood that was almost idiomatically popular in early modern Europe. Russians certainly used this procedure, including on the royal family, but the oath does not mention it.[7] Bloodletting is associated with the controversial practice of astrology, as bleeding must occur on the correct day. Medical astrology was debated at the Russian court, but its usage was not prescribed or proscribed in the oath.[8] Apothecary Chancery practitioners also gave advice, a key part of early modern medicine, yet the giving of advice is also not mentioned.[9] Surgery, a vital yet hazardous activity, receives one perfunctory phrase in one manuscript of the oath.[10] Drugs, on the other hand, receive substantial attention in every extant copy. Among the various hazards of medical treatment that the Apothecary Chancery could have concerned itself in its oath, it chose specifically to focus on medical drugs.

Also significant is the issue of who was swearing to carefully construct medical drugs. The Apothecary Chancery employed multiple groups of people. On the administrative side, there was the director, a high-ranking Russian noble [*boiar*].[11] He was assisted by a committee of junior directors [*sud'i* pl., *sud'ia* sing.], usually career administrators known as secretaries [*d'iaki* pl., *d'iak* sing.], who would advise the head director how to proceed. Under this committee of directors worked a number of other secretaries and undersecretaries [*pod'iachie* pl., *pod'iachii* sing.].[12] The department also employed translators, to facilitate communication between the mostly Russian administrators and the primarily non-Russian medical staff.

Within the medical staff of the department, there were also multiple distinctions, of duties, responsibilities, and salaries. The highest rank of medical practitioner in the Apothecary Chancery was that of physician [pl. *dokhtury, dokhtur* sing.], a rank typically occupied by a university-educated foreign physician. Senior physicians could be paid up to 1,114r per annum; junior physicians were commonly paid 460r per annum.[13] Their boss, the head of the department, was paid at least one-third more than the physicians; his state secretaries [*dumnye d'iaki* pl.; *dumnyi d'iak* sing.] earned a similar salary to that of the physicians.[14] In broader context, physicians' wages were similar to that earned by middling court ranks like a military governor [*voevoda*], an arms bearer [*okol'nichii*], or a steward [*stol'nik*]. Aside from the nobles, the only groups earning substantially more than the senior physicians were some other foreign experts, as well as generals.[15] The physicians then were compensated similarly to some of their senior chancery colleagues, but less than both their immediate superior and certain of their neighbours in the foreigners' quarter of Moscow.

Beneath the physicians in the medical ranks were the apothecaries [*aptekari* pl., *aptekar'* sing.], typically trained in Western European guilds. The apothecaries worked with assistants, the alchemists [*alkhemisty* pl., *alkhemist* sing.] and distillers [*distiliatory* pl., *distiliator* sing.].[16] Pay for the distillers was typically between 110 and 130 rubles per annum; apothecaries received more, between 140 and 360 rubles per annum, but substantially less than the top physicians.[17] Not only were they paid less than the physicians and the state secretaries, they were paid less than other Russian colleagues like the secretaries and clerks as well as the interpreters and translators.[18] This then put them in a similar salary range to military ranks like a captain or a *ratnyi chelovek* [lit. military person], middling administrators like a secretary, a clerk, or a local artisan like a blacksmith.[19] The apothecaries were then positioned alongside other servitors with useful skills but who were not leaders or advisers.

Lowest of the Apothecary Chancery's permanent medical staff were the surgical ranks. This included surgeons [*lekari* pl., *lekar'* sing.] and field surgeons [*polevye lekari* pl., *polevoi lekar'* sing.], as well as specialists like bone setters [*kostopravy* pl., *kostoprav* sing.]. Their pay was the lowest of all the Apothecary Chancery medical ranks: 50 rubles per annum was a typical salary for these men, although they could receive as much as

140 rubles per annum.[20] Their typical salary is then comparable to that of a bailiff, a musketeer, a sergeant, or a provincial servitor.[21] Pay-wise, the surgeons were bracketed with lower-middle military and court ranks.

From 1654 on, the Apothecary Chancery also had apothecary and surgery pupils, men usually taken from the musketeers' ranks who were apprenticed to a foreign practitioner. Their pay reflected their position at the bottom of the ranks: the lowest-paid pupils were paid an official salary of just 1 ruble per annum. Pay to Apothecary Chancery staff included both this yearly salary and a monthly payment. Combining these, the lowest-paid pupil in the 1650s received 10 rubles 32 *altyn* for the year's work. After pay rises in the early 1660s, a pupil could then receive as much as 29 rubles per annum.[22] This was an incredibly modest salary, putting them below all other employees of the department, including the guards who protected the building they worked in.[23] Pupils, then, were very low down in the economic stratification of the Muscovite service ranks.

We can see who from these groups of administrative and medical personnel took the oaths by looking at those documents themselves. All such oaths end with the phrase "I attach my signature" [lit. hand], followed by the servitor's signature. Symbolically, this shows the total acceptance of the precepts of the oath by the oath taker. Pragmatically, it also tells us who took the oath. Evidence from oaths across the seventeenth century shows apothecaries and physicians, surgeons, and even translators, all taking the same oath: one manuscript lists the apothecary Roman and the surgeons Matvei and Elisarei as all swearing the same oath; another the translators Matvei Eliseev, Vasilii Oleksandrov, and Andrei (no surname listed), as well as the surgeon Samoil Kam.[24] Employees directly involved with making drugs, such as the apothecaries, employees responsible for prescribing drugs like the physicians, and even employees with no role in the creation of drugs like the translators, all took an oath declaring that they would be careful in the creation of drugs.

This insistence that all staff in the department take an oath relating to the creation of drugs is unusual. To see just how unusual, we need to look at medical oaths of this period more broadly. The history of medical oaths in early modern Western Europe, from which the Apothecary Chancery took much of its medical practices, is less well researched than one might expect. Nevertheless, certain general points can be established. The most famous such text is the Hippocratic Oath, an ancient world text derived from the Hippocratic corpus of works associated with the ancient Greek physician Hippocrates of Kos, although the oath is one of several texts in the Hippocratic corpus that are unlikely to have been written by Hippocrates himself. The version of the Hippocratic Oath that is used in some medical schools today is also different from the original. Moreover, there is a significant historical gap between the composition of this text in ancient Greece and its modern-day use; there is only one definitive recording of it being used in early modern Europe, in Wittenberg, Germany, in 1508.[25] Instead, multiple medical bodies in multiple polities wrote their own oaths.[26]

Looking more closely at these early modern Western European medical oaths, we see important differences from Apothecary Chancery procedures. In the documents of the Royal College Of Medicine and Public Health of Brandenburg-Prussia (est. 1685), physicians swore not to make their own medicines, other than secret preparations not available in pharmacies, but to use a trusted – and licensed – apothecary.[27] A mid-fifteenth-century town physician oath from Amberg, southern Germany, set down broadly the same rules, as did a 1601 regulation for Frankfurt am Main in western Germany.[28] Similarly, an eighteenth-century German oath required the physician to oversee pharmacies, but not to take an active part in making drugs.[29] Here we see a minimization of the role of physicians in drug creation. In stark contrast to the Apothecary Chancery oaths, which made all medical practitioners take responsibility for drugs, the oaths for physicians from the early modern German lands see little role for these medical practitioners in the creation of drugs. Indeed, they often take the opposite approach, requiring physicians to keep their distance from the drug-creation processes.

The real details about drug creation in Western Europe come from the oaths specifically aimed at the properly enfranchised drug creators: the apothecaries. Returning to the Royal College of Medicine and Public Health of Brandenburg-Prussia, we see that it set down many such rules for the apothecaries it licensed: not to sell without the approval or foreknowledge of a physician any purgatives, emetics, diuretics, or opiates, much less poisons.[30] The fifteenth-century pharmacy oath from Amberg required the taker to swear to keep his medicines well, protect them from mice, and to take particular care of any potentially harmful medicines.[31] The 1601 law from Frankfurt am Main required apothecaries to swear an oath on the good quality and suitability of medicines in their pharmacy.[32] Seventeenth- and eighteenth-century Dutch pharmacy oaths from

Leeuwarden, Leiden, and Den Haag all lay down similar conditions: adhering to the regulations of the guild and the pharmacopoeia, stocking the correct ingredients, preparing medicines according to physicians' prescriptions, and selling poisonous goods with caution.[33] A model oath, written in Latin in 1608, translated into French in 1637, and in use in some French regions in the mid-seventeenth century, makes a number of comments on making drugs, including a pledge to consult a physician before prescribing or making substitutions, and to promise not to stock bad drugs, not to give poison to anyone, nor help anyone to give poison to another.[34] Western European medical institutions then set out careful and detailed rules regarding the proper creation, storage, and use of medical drugs and the central place of the apothecary in those processes.

We can then see the Apothecary Chancery oath as expressing a very specific viewpoint on the role of medical drugs in official Russian medical culture. The creation of medical drugs was considered important and potentially dangerous above even other kinds of medical practice engaged in by the department. All employees of the department had to take the oath, regardless of their role in the creation of drugs, again underlining its centrality to the work of the department. Moreover, this practice of focusing so heavily on medical drugs and on having all employees take the same oath substantially deviates from the various contemporary oaths of Western Europe, which tend to separate out the work of medical practitioners in their oaths. Beginning with the Apothecary Chancery oath, we can already see the focus on medical drugs as particularly, perhaps even uniquely, important to the Russian context.

PROTECTING THE TSAR

The Apothecary Chancery oath then shows notable departures from other contemporary medical oaths. Indeed, there is reason to consider the Apothecary Chancery oath, and its particular emphasis on medical drugs, from a different perspective. The Apothecary Chancery took a substantial amount of their official medical world from Western Europe: practitioners, books, equipment, ingredients, even words; the very names of the department across the sixteenth and seventeenth centuries – *Aptechnaia izba, Aptekarskii prikaz* – were taken in part from the Western European term "apothecary." And so we must consider the Apothecary Chancery oaths in the context of Western European oaths. But we also need to put those oaths in the other vital context from which that text sprung: Muscovy. Fundamentally, the Apothecary Chancery oath was Muscovite. It was a medical practice oath, but it was also an oath of service, from a culture with a long history of service and loyalty oaths. Putting these medical oaths side by side with other Muscovite oaths we see that this focus on medical drugs was something that sprung more from Muscovite culture than Western European medical practice.

The text of the oath raises questions as to the relationship of the medical oaths of the Apothecary Chancery to other Muscovite service oaths. In some respects, the concerns of the Apothecary Chancery oath over drugs were not entirely medical. The text specifies that drugs must not spoil [*isportit', s porcheiu*] a patient. Although this term "spoiling" did have a broader usage, it was most commonly associated with witchcraft. As for the banned drugs themselves, they are referred to as evil [*likhii*], and as unclean in a ritual sense [*nichistii*]. The term cunning [*khitrii, khitrost'*], used in the Apothecary Chancery oath to describe unwanted and inappropriate behaviours, was also associated with witchcraft.[35] According to Valerie Kivelson, poisoning was commonly linked to witchcraft.[36] The essence of this link was that conflation of powerful consumed items and their ability to do harm in the Russian word *zel'ia*, repeatedly used in the Apothecary Chancery oaths. Practitioners taking the Apothecary Chancery oath were not only agreeing to abide by rules relating to correct pharmaceutical practices, they were simultaneously swearing off the practices of poisoning and malefic magic.

Such concerns over both witchcraft and poisoning also appear in boyars' oaths, the oaths taken by Russian nobles making up the tsar's close retinue who played a key role in the Russian bureaucracy, including heading up departments such as the Apothecary Chancery. From at least 1598, and certainly throughout the seventeenth century, these oaths required the taker to abstain from bewitching or poisoning the tsar.[37] Indeed, these oaths use the very same terms also used in the Apothecary Chancery oaths. The culture complex that put together poison-potion-medicine, combined with the fear of poisoning at court, indicates the origin of the Apothecary Chancery's particular concern with medical drugs. The Apothecary Chancery oath's extensive concern with this issue was a modification and amplification of the concern over poison, heightened in an atmosphere in which consumable medicines were a fundamental part of healing.

The Apothecary Chancery oath was also linked to other Muscovite oaths by the injunction to watch colleagues and report their misbehaviours. Muscovite service oaths commonly included what Ann Kleimola has dubbed the "duty to denounce" – promises to report the illicit behaviour of others.[38] A key concern of these oaths was the duty of Muscovite servitors to safeguard their sovereign, commonly by denouncing anyone they heard plotting against the tsar.[39] Some of these oaths, in particular those from the turbulent years at the start of the seventeenth century, mentioned poisoning specifically as a plot needing to be reported. This duty to denounce binds the Apothecary Chancery oaths to contemporary Muscovite service oaths.

During the period in which the Apothecary Chancery functioned, there was indeed reason to be concerned over such political plots and poisonings. In 1584, Tsar Ivan IV died after a turbulent and often violent reign. This sparked theories, both at the time and more recently, that he may have been murdered. Following Ivan's passing, his youngest son Dmitrii died under suspicious circumstances in 1591 and his elder son Fedor I died in 1598 without fathering any children. Fedor's one-time regent Boris Godunov formally took the throne, and the country slid into the period of dynastic crisis known as the Time of Troubles. This short period – the start of which is dated to either Fedor's death in 1598 or to Godunov's in 1605, and the end to 1613 with the election of Mikhail Fedorovich as the first tsar of the new Romanov dynasty – saw many more suspicious deaths and rumoured poisonings. Such poisoning accusations continued into the Romanov period, with Mikhail Fedorovich's first fiancée Maria Khlopova suffering from a stomach ailment in 1616 possibly caused by poisoning.[40] We can connect these poisoning rumours to court medicine via the figure of Eliseus Bomelius. Bomelius worked as a medical practitioner at the Russian court in the 1570s, but was also rumoured to have worked as a poisoner for Ivan IV until the latter had Bomelius executed for disloyalty in 1579; those rumours took on a theatrical afterlife as Bomelius appears as the villain in N.A. Rimsky-Korsakov's 1898 opera *The Tsar's Bride*.[41] The Moscow court had good reason to fear poisonings, both from members of court and from medical practitioners.

The duty to denounce that was used in the sixteenth and seventeenth centuries to attempt to guard against poisonings had a longer textual history. As established by Ann Kleimola, Muscovite service oaths ultimately derive from fourteenth-century inter-princely agreements. The latter were not service oaths, although they were, in a way, loyalty oaths: each prince pledged to be true to the other in their agreements. Particularly significantly, the requirement to denounce to the prince plots against him is also found in the inter-princely agreements; each party pledged to inform the other of political moves made against them.[42] The Apothecary Chancery oath was then in some senses closer to the practices of medieval East Slavic diplomacy than it was to early modern Western European medicine.

Mukharji, Slater, López-Terrada, and Pardo-Tomás all emphasize that medical practices were bound up with other aspects of contemporary society, politics, religion, and culture. This is certainly true of the Apothecary Chancery oaths. They were one variation on the ever-present Muscovite service oath, sharing those documents' concerns over *zel'ia*; through them we can trace the concerns in the department's oaths back to earlier documents that inspired the Muscovite oaths. The imprecation of the Apothecary Chancery oath against badly created medicines was part of a longer concern over bewitchment, poisoning, and betrayal that can be traced back to fourteenth-century East Slavic diplomacy.

INTERNAL AFFAIRS

As we can see from their oath, the Apothecary Chancery was always concerned about the correct practice of creating medical drugs. Other Apothecary Chancery documents show that those strict rules on preparing medicines were in fact applied in a number of internal disciplinary cases, in particular in the late seventeenth century. Interestingly, although there were concerns over witchcraft and poisoning at court in this period, the internal Apothecary Chancery investigations discussed infractions within the narrow confines of medical malpractice. The standards of behaviour set out in the Apothecary Chancery oath were taken from long-term East Slavic concerns over poisoning and bewitching, but within the department bad behaviour was more narrowly defined in terms of questionable medical practice. Yet the connection remained: internal investigations in the Apothecary Chancery were concerned specifically with medical drugs.

The first place we can see traces of how the oath worked is in the format of Apothecary Chancery prescriptions. Prescriptions record the ingredients put into a medicine, to whom it was given, and usually also who made up the medicine and who prescribed it. They were drafted in Latin, as it was the foreign physicians who decided what medicines were to be made and the foreign apothecaries who were to make it, and Latin was the lingua franca of the Western European medical practitioners in the department. It was then translated into Russian, so that the Russian bureaucrats could also see what had been prescribed and created, by whom, and for whom. Interesting here is what is typically absent from these documents: the majority of such prescriptions do not state what ailment they are to treat. This then indicates the purpose of Apothecary Chancery prescriptions. They are not about what to treat, they are about who to blame. In the context of a department where medical practitioners had to take responsibility for the contents and effects of medicines, the prescriptions were one way in which that responsibility could be tracked.

The department made use of those records of responsibility: a number of documents testify to internal investigations into the preparation of medicines. Most such transgressions appear to have been relatively minor: in 1673 a member of staff incorrectly measured the quantities of water added to concentrated medicines before sale in the Apothecary Chancery's Moscow shop in which ordinary Muscovites could purchase medical drugs; in 1685 two Apothecary Chancery auxiliary staff members stole departmental supplies to make gin, violating the Russian state's monopoly on the production of distilled alcohol as well as committing a theft of government property.[43] Most significantly here, also in 1685 a staff member called Kuz'ma Dmitriev accidentally substituted a phial of water for one of essence of rosemary.[44] This is exactly the kind of infraction the Apothecary Chancery oath specifically spoke against, in this case an accidental replacement of a correct medicine with an incorrect one. Dmitriev's actions were not discussed as malicious, but they were nevertheless strictly forbidden. Despite the minor nature of these infractions, and the fact that no one was hurt by them, the defendants in all cases were sentenced to corporal punishment. Throughout the seventeenth century, the creation of Apothecary Chancery remedies was carefully monitored, and infractions punished, just as laid out in the departmental oath.

More serious cases in which Apothecary Chancery practitioners were investigated for potentially causing harm were less common. In 1682 an Apothecary Chancery physician, Arnold van der Hulst, was suspected of causing the death of his patient, Fedor Neledinskii. As a result, the Apothecary Chancery opened an investigation, beginning with three questions: from what illness had Neledinskii been suffering; which medicines had van der Hulst given him; and what was the cause of Neledinskii's death? The department also required van der Hulst to provide a list of medicines he had prescribed to Neledinskii. From the start of the investigation, the department focused on medical drugs, rather than asking about van der Hulst's treatment of Neledinskii as a whole.

Having received the prescription records from van der Hulst, the department then instructed a fellow Apothecary Chancery physician, Andrei Kellerman, to perform an autopsy on the deceased. Kellerman was specifically asked to examine certain marks on the body and determine if they had been caused by the medical drugs prescribed by van der Hulst. Kellerman concluded that there were no signs on the body to indicate that Neledinskii died from the medical drugs given to him by van der Hulst, but rather that death had resulted from the fever for which van Hulst had been treating him.[45] There are any number of points on which a physician could be questioned after the death of a patient. Yet once again, in this case the explicit focus of the Apothecary Chancery's concerns were the medicines van der Hulst had prescribed.

These concerns extended into the eighteenth century. In 1703, the Apothecary Chancery apothecary Daniel Gurchin was investigated for incorrectly preparing *confectio alkermes* (also known as *confectio alchermes*); this medicine was a well-known Arabic herbal concoction given to those with weak hearts.[46] Gurchin was accused by his colleague, and one-time collaborator on the *Domestic and Field Pharmacy*, Laurentius Blumentrost senior. During the investigation, another Apothecary Chancery medical practitioner, the alchemist Peter Pil, also denounced Gurchin's work.[47] The key here was the identification of the *kermes* – commonly referred to, as it is in these document, as a seed, but actually a small insect, the *Coccus ilicis* – central to the production of this medicine. Gurchin claimed he had the correct seed; his colleagues contradicted him. Eventually, the opinion of Blumentrost and Pil was upheld, and Gurchin was ordered to use the seeds for his own purposes, and not to sell them. The concern over substituting ingredients in medicines explicitly voiced by the Apothecary Chancery oath at the start of the seventeenth century was still an issue within the department by the start of the eighteenth century.

The Apothecary Chancery oaths, and the earlier documents on which they are based, present an ideal state of affairs, a set of rules and a code of conduct stating how people should behave. Looking at records of how people did behave within the department, we see a clear reflection of the major concern of the Apothecary Chancery oath. In the period for which we have good records of internal medical malpractice investigations within the department, the 1670s–1700s, those investigations are narrowly concerned with the correct creation of medical drugs and the potential effects of those drugs on the human body, responsibility for which was placed upon the medical staff who prescribed and created those drugs. The Apothecary Chancery's concern with medical drugs went beyond the theoretical behaviours set out in the oath and had a real impact on the running of the department.

POLICING THE MARKETPLACE

This concern with medical drugs that was encoded in the Apothecary Chancery oath and expressed in the internal investigations also shaped the department's role in the broader regulation of medicine in the Russian Empire. Across the course of the seventeenth century the Apothecary Chancery was increasingly involved in cases against those accused of using natural objects for witchcraft or medical malpractice. These two groups of cases are often treated separately as they fall into distinct categories of modern research, history of magic, and history of medicine. Yet the process and details of these cases show that they had much in common, following a shared pattern in which another part of the chancery system began proceedings against the accused on the basis of their ownership or usage of a natural object, and the Apothecary Chancery was then asked to give an expert opinion on the properties of that object. The medical culture of the Apothecary Chancery that centred on medical drugs was a part of a broader interest in the powers of natural objects within the Russian Empire, and that connection underpinned the department's entrance into policing the medical marketplace.

The earliest witchcraft case in which the Apothecary Chancery was asked to play a role occurred in 1628, when a suspicious root was found in the possession of the peasant Andrei Loptunov. This case is significant, as many of its features are echoed in later documents concerning the Apothecary Chancery's involvement in witchcraft trials. When questioned about the herb found on him, Loptunov stated that "the root he had wrapped around a crucifix was given to him by a passer-by on the road, and from which town [this man came] he does not know, and [the man] gave him that root because Andrei suffers from epilepsy [lit. black illness]."[48] Andrei's claims were partly corroborated by his master, Mikhail Polibin, who stated that Loptunov had been released from service to travel to places of veneration [*po sviatym mestam*] in search of a cure for his illness.

Having heard Loptunov's testimony, and that of his master, the court decided on further tests of Andrei's story, and his characterization of the root as medicinal, by sending the root to the Apothecary Chancery for examination. As the report states,

> And the root that was taken from the peasant Andrei Loptunov was shown to the doctors in the Apothecary Chamber.[49] And Doctor Valentine [Bills] and his colleagues, having looked at the root, said that this root [is called] Goose-flesh, and is used in medicines, and has nothing evil in it, and [people] put that root in the mouth. And if someone wished to commit a crime, and [if] he used the good herb badly, for criminality or witchcraft, that they do not know, [and they do not know] if there is a curse on that root.[50]

This focus on the root in the investigation is significant. The need to establish the root's properties suggests that the root could have certain inherent qualities as a natural object that would particularly recommend it for witchcraft; essentially, that a root could be magical. This demonstrates that the Russian authorities were concerned with the root itself, not the circumstances under which it was obtained.

The name of Loptunov's plant – Goose-flesh – is also significant. As an illogical reference to an animal to name an herb, it follows a general pattern of Slavic names for local herbs. Local herbs frequently appear in the witchcraft trials. In 1664 the *syn boyarskii* Dmitrii Volodemirov was found to have suspicious herbs with him when he was searched at the Patriarch's palace. These herbs were examined in the Apothecary Chancery, with the following report written on the results: "[there are] the herb *karniana*, another herb *kanisa*, and they said that those herbs are field herbs[51] and nothing bad will come of those herbs, and they cannot identify [lit. know] the other herbs as those herbs have been chopped up."[52] The concern over herbs as *materia magica* was also a concern over the potentially harmful nature of local plants.

Russian witchcraft trials, including those sent to the Apothecary Chancery, commonly related to local plants, the same category of natural object that the department relied upon in creating medicines. As Loptunov did in 1628, many of those accused in the witchcraft trials claimed that the items found on them were *materia medica*, not *materia magica.* Sometimes the overlap between the medically useful and the magically criminal was even greater: in one case, a plant presented as evidence in a witchcraft trial was simultaneously in use in the Apothecary Chancery, the same department to which the potentially magical plant had been sent for assessment. The Apothecary Chancery report from that 1657 witchcraft case states

> And in the Apothecary Chancery the doctors and apothecaries, examining the roots, said that the root was *bolderian* [valerian] and from that root nothing bad occurs, and the other root they cannot identify [lit. know], as it [the root] has dried up and they have no essence, and so nothing bad can come from these roots and of those roots [they] identified one root and called [it] *bolderian* and for what that root is used they did not say.[53]

Valerian root was a well-known medicinal substance in the early modern world: Nicholas Culpeper included a chapter on it when he wrote his *Complete Herbal* in 1653.[54] More locally, it was discussed as a medicinal substance in the Apothecary Chancery only a few years after this case: in 1665, the department produced a report on it including material from Latin-language and Russian-language sources.[55] Valerian root was then one item that balanced on the narrow precipice between approved medicament and outlawed *materia magica*.

Apothecary Chancery involvement in witchcraft trials continued into the later seventeenth century and even the eighteenth century. The department did not take part in all the Russian witchcraft trials, but they regularly took part in them from the 1620s to the 1700s.[56] The involvement of the department in such trials was sufficiently well known by the end of the century that one defendant in a trial in 1690 specifically asked for the herbs that had been found on him to be examined by the department, as he believed their testimony would exonerate him by supporting his claim that the herbs were medicinal.[57]

In the second half of the seventeenth century, the Apothecary Chancery applied the same procedures they had been using in witchcraft trials to medical malpractice investigations. Notably, this did not involve churchmen. We know that Russian Orthodox churchmen continued their religious healing practices in this period, but although that was an extra-departmental practice it was still licit.[58] Rather, the department was increasingly engaged in investigating secular, unofficial medical practitioners. This almost always revolved around consumable medicines. The knowledge of the Apothecary

Chancery experts, which could be used to create good medicines for the courtly elite or adjudicate in witchcraft trials, could also be used to identify bad medicines provided to the denizens of Moscow.

In some cases, the Apothecary Chancery became involved in irregular medical practice because of a clash between official and unofficial medical practitioners. In 1652, the Apothecary Chancery surgeon Andrei Ivanov brought a case against the unofficial practitioner Dmitrii Selunskii. Ivanov and Selunskii had both treated the same patient, Semyon Korobin, who had later died because, Ivanov claimed, Selunskii had given the man an inappropriate medicament.[59] Such hiring of multiple practitioners was common in early modern medicine and frequently led to conflicts between rival practitioners.[60] In part the 1652 Selunskii case is about the right to practise.

It was also about practice and malpractice. Central to Ivanov's case against Selunskii was his accusation that the latter had prescribed Korobin opium, a medicament Ivanov claimed would not have helped Korobin's condition. Opium, famous in the modern world as a potent medicinal and recreational drug, is perhaps surprisingly rare in early modern Russian drug documents. Poppies, the botanical origin of the processed medicament opium, do appear regularly in official Russian medical documents.[61] But opium itself appears only twice in Apothecary Chancery prescriptions.[62] Opium, then, could be used as a medicine, but was not appropriate for Korobin, and so Selunskii, in Ivanov's view, had committed medical malpractice by prescribing incorrect medicines. The interrogation of Selunskii then focused on this central issue of what he prescribed, even as he also admitted to treating wounds and bleeding patients.[63] As early as 1652, the Apothecary Chancery was specifically focused upon consumable medicines as a key issue in malpractice investigations of the broader medical marketplace.

Ivanov and Selunskii ended up treating the same patient in 1652 because Korobin had hired them both. Members of court who had the right to Apothecary Chancery treatment sometimes also combined this with unofficial practitioners. Indeed, no less a figure than the former Apothecary Chancery director boyar Boris Ivanovich Morozov used both the Apothecary Chancery physician Samuel Collins and an unofficial medical practitioner then in his service during his final illness in 1661.[64] Morozov's death, like that of Ivanov and Selunskii's patient, was also investigated by the Apothecary Chancery. Again, it was this overlap between the spheres of official and unofficial medicine created by patient-consumers that seem to have occasioned the investigation.

Similar to the Selunskii case, the investigation quickly focused on the consumable medicines the unofficial practitioner provided. This practitioner, Fedor Belozertsov, was questioned in particular about his provision to Morozov of the herb *zaiach'e kopyto,* literally hare's hoof, another plant named using the typically deliberately illogical folk naming system for plants with special uses.[65] Belozertsov stated that he had acquired this herb on Morozov's insistence, as a treatment for *mokrotnaia bolezn'* [phlegmatic illness]. Belozertsov also stated that he had previously given the same hare's hoof herb to his mother, who had then lived for a further twenty years.[66] As Kirill Khudin has demonstrated, figures like Belozertsov reveal how healing formed a nexus connecting multiple different groups in Muscovite society, from nobles to court doctors to unofficial practitioners; it was this nexus that led to the Apothecary Chancery's increasing interest in individual cases of unofficial medicine.[67]

The medical culture of the Apothecary Chancery was internally consistent, with both oaths and internal investigations focusing on medical drugs. That focus can also be seen in other doctoring traditions of the Russian Empire, with practices coded by Russian officials and scholars as magical healing or unofficial secular medical practice both using natural objects, often consumable natural objects, as a central part of those traditions. This shared belief in the centrality of consuming natural objects for changing the state of the human body led to the Apothecary Chancery's role in both witchcraft trials and medical malpractice trials. Medical drugs can be most easily traced in the Apothecary Chancery as that department left us so many documents, but reading the trial records of other practitioners shows that the department shared that concern with others in the Russian Empire. There was, to borrow language from Mukharji, a common strand of concern with medical drugs that was braided into both official and unofficial doctoring traditions of the Russian Empire, and so led to the increasing encroachment of the official into the realm of the unofficial.

MISSION CREEP

From the 1620s on the Apothecary Chancery applied the concerns about natural objects it had inherited from earlier East Slavic documents to participating in witchcraft trials; from the 1650s it applied the procedures developed in those witchcraft trials to individual cases of medical malpractice originating outside of the department. As the seventeenth century wore on, those individual cases led the Moscow authorities to make larger-scale investigations into the practice of unofficial medicine. These investigations, taking place in the 1680s and 1690s, particularly focused on the sales of medicines and medical ingredients on the Kitai-gorod markets and would in turn spark a broader regulation of unofficial medicines. The specific concern over a group of objects into which consumable medicines fell had consequences not only for the court where the Apothecary Chancery practised, but also for Muscovite society more generally.

As with the cases against individual unofficial practitioners from the 1650s and 1660s, the death of important people also played a role in sparking the broader investigations of the final decades of the seventeenth century. In 1679, Prince Fedor Shcherbatskii died after taking medicines purchased on the Kitai-gorod markets, a central trading region of Moscow.[68] This case is similar to the medical malpractice cases from earlier in the century in that it revolved again around the key issue of medical drugs and was arbitrated by the Apothecary Chancery. Yet the Shcherbatskii case also included two new features that would fuel later investigations.

The first novel feature was that the investigation into Shcherbatskii's death was not initiated by an Apothecary Chancery practitioner, as had previously been the case, but rather by a civilian, Iurii Shcherbatskii, the brother of the deceased. Moreover, he did not approach the department itself. Instead, Iurii Shcherbatskii approached the Musketeers' Chancery with his claim of malpractice against the man he believed responsible for his brother's death, Grigorii Donskoi. It was only then that the Apothecary Chancery became involved, on the request of the Musketeers' Chancery. The key role played by two groups from outside the Apothecary Chancery – the Shcherbatskii family and the Musketeers' Chancery – changed the nature of the investigation. The 1679 case was not an issue of an Apothecary Chancery practitioner making accusations against one specific competitor, but of the Muscovite elite drawing multiple departments into an investigation.

The second novel feature was how this investigation proceeded within the department. As with the earlier cases, the focus was on consumable medicines. According to his brother, after taking Donskoi's medicine Fedor Shcherbatskii had developed sores in his mouth, become sicker, and died shortly thereafter. The remaining medicine was sent to the

Apothecary Chancery, where it was subject to not one but two different examinations; in both cases the examination was focused on establishing the contents of the medicine, which were suspected to include mercury. The foreign physicians who initially examined the medicine could not give a clear answer on the issue. A group of Russian surgeons then identified most but not all of the ingredients; crucially, they were unable to definitively say whether it contained mercury. This investigation then involved the family of the deceased, the Musketeers' Chancery, and two different groups of medical practitioners from within the Apothecary Chancery. Although the Shcherbatskii investigation of 1679 was focused on one incident, it was beginning to take on the sprawling nature that would be typical of later investigations.

This case-by-case investigation of irregular practice typified by the cases against Selunskii, Belozertsov, and Donskoi in the 1650s–70s coalesced into a more structured inquiry into unofficial *materia medica* in the final decades of the seventeenth century. In 1685, the Apothecary Chancery undertook an investigation into the sale of one particular medicine. The head of the Musketeers' Chancery was then scrutinizing the activities of the herbal stalls [*zelenyi riad*] in the Kitai-gorod markets, and wanted to know if a certain herb – identified in all documents simply as the "heady herb" [*p'ianoe zel'ia*] – was approved for use as an internal medicine, and if a licence was required to sell it.[69] Apothecary Chancery experts declared the "heady herb" unfit for use in internal medicine after an examination of texts in the Apothecary Chancery library revealed that it was not listed as medicinal.[70] The report further added that the "heady herb" was dangerous, capable of causing amnesia [*zabvenie uma*], and even death.[71] Here we begin to see mission creep, as the rules of the Apothecary Chancery were increasingly applied to medical practice beyond the walls of that institution.

The investigations of a chemical medicine in 1679 and an herbal medicine in 1685 were both centred on one specific Moscow region: Kitai-gorod. Kitai-gorod was the major trading region of Moscow throughout the sixteenth and seventeenth centuries, located just to the east of both the Kremlin and Red Square. By the time of the Kitai-gorod investigations, the Apothecary Chancery building was no longer in the Kremlin proper, but just outside the walls to the northwest, by the Trinity Tower entrance to the Kremlin. The building still stands today, located on Starovagankovskii pereulok just behind the Leninka library, which now holds some of the older institution's treasured texts. Anyone familiar with Moscow's urban geography will know how close all those buildings are. The transgressing market holders were then peddling their wares only a few minutes' walk away from the centre of government and the major official medical department of the empire.

The problems with the Kitai-gorod markets came to a head in 1699–1700, when the Apothecary Chancery again began an investigation of the medicines being sold there. That investigation, like those in 1679 and 1685, was sparked by the death of a member of the elite, boyar P.P. Saltykov, following the consumption of medicines from those markets.[72] Unlike those earlier investigations, which had focused on specific transgressors, as in 1679, or on the sale of one herb, as in 1685, in 1699–1700 the inquiry broadened into a general survey of all merchants selling medical drugs on the Kitai-gorod markets and what they sold. By 1699 it was no longer a case of isolated incidents being dealt with one by one, but a concerted government effort to investigate and punish an entire group of medical practitioners, the stallholders of the Moscow markets.

During the investigation six Kitai-gorod stallholders were interrogated in the Apothecary Chancery. The testimony of all six is markedly similar: all admitted to stocking some medical supplies, including ointments [*mazi*] and plasters, but specifically denied selling internal medicines [*vnutrennye lekarstva*]. As the only female stallholder said, "internal medicines and any other [such medicines] and oils she, Agrofenka [Leont'eva], does not stock".[73] As this testimony was shaped by the bureaucrats asking the questions, the physicians assisting them, and the scribes recording the answers, this division between internal medicines and externally applied treatments like plasters and ointments came from the Apothecary Chancery itself.[74] Indeed, we can see this focus on internal medicines in earlier legislation. The 1673 decree establishing the New Pharmacy also outlined the exclusive right of that branch of the Apothecary Chancery to sell internal medicines.[75] The testimony of Leont'eva and her fellow stallholders was then an implicit response to the officially proscribed limits of their trade as defined in 1673: they were permitted to sell some healing products, but not the more concerning internal medicines.

The 1699–1700 investigation was focused on the Kitai-gorod merchants, but it affected a broader system of unofficial practice. One of Leont'eva's competitors, the trader Vasilii Kirilov, stated that he stocked his stall from items brought to him by rural people who collected plants in the fields near where they lived.[76] Although Kirilov was the one being interrogated, the disruption to his market trade would have meant a disruption to the livelihood of these villagers, too. The work of medical practitioners like Leont'eva, Kirilov, and their unnamed suppliers often only enter the written historical record in investigations like this; the use of the Apothecary Chancery expertise to investigate the broader world of medical practice in late seventeenth-century Moscow reveals to us an ecosystem of unofficial medical practice just as those investigations were disrupting it. And those investigations show that, like the Apothecary Chancery itself, unofficial medical practice was also substantially concerned with medical drugs.

The nature of the Russian situation, in which unofficial practitioners rarely if ever kept written records and the official department kept substantial records, means that our view of the doctoring traditions of the early modern Russian Empire will always be skewed towards the concerns of official medicine. Yet through that official lens we can see something of unofficial practice as it came into contact and conflict with officialdom. We do not know the full extent of the activities of Selunskii, Belozertsov, Donskoi, Leont'eva, and Kirilov, and so their work may have included a variety of practices unknown to us. Yet we do know that their doctoring traditions were braided together with official practices by a common interest in medical drugs, and it was the use of those drugs that brought them to the attention of the Apothecary Chancery. Inasmuch as we can know anything about the unofficial medical practitioners of the early modern Russian Empire, we do know that they shared the Apothecary Chancery's interest in medical drugs.

CONCLUSION

Beginning this book on *materia medica* gives us the opportunity to understand why that focus is particularly appropriate to the study of early modern Russian medicine. We can do so by considering what Mukharji called "doctoring traditions" and what Slater, López-Terrada, and Pardo-Tomás call "medical cultures": the specific nature of medical practices in the early modern Russian Empire. As we have seen in this chapter, both official and unofficial medical practice in early modern Russia, as well as linked but distinct traditions like court culture and witchcraft, all saw consumable natural objects – medical drugs – as uniquely powerful in affecting the human body. This book, then, is about *materia medica* because that was the central aspect of early modern Russian medical practice.

That central aspect is most clearly expressed in official texts, medical documents, and court documents. The Apothecary Chancery oath directly states that medical drugs are a key concern of the department, a precept put into practice multiple times in the department's internal investigations. That concern with the specific category of medical drugs can be traced to the fear of the broader category of *zel'ia* [poison-potion-drug] in other Muscovite service oaths, and from there as far back as fourteenth-century East Slavic Princely agreements. Officials in Muscovy had a specific concern over the power of natural objects to affect the human body. This concern tied together poisons, potions, and medicines into one concept that could be either the most helpful thing for the human body, or the deadliest. Understandably then, Muscovite officials spent more time constructing and applying rules and procedures to control the production and use of medical drugs than they did any other branch of medicine. The history of the Apothecary Chancery is largely the history of its drug-making and drug-regulating procedures.

That fundamental concern also reveals how and why official medicine came into contact and conflict with unofficial medical practitioners, both those prosecuted as medical practitioners and those prosecuted as magical practitioners. The nature of these trials, which commonly revolved around the properties and usage of natural objects and their effects on the human body, shows that unofficial medicine also held a substantial place for medical drugs. We cannot see the entirety of unofficial practice from these documents; there may have been other significant aspects of those practices not discussed in the investigations. But we can see that there was a substantial overlap between official and unofficial medicine on the issue of medical drugs. We can return here to thinking about strands of different doctoring traditions being braided more closely together or unravelling from each other. We do not know all the strands that made up unofficial medical practice in the early modern Russian Empire, but we know that one strand was medical drugs, and that bound unofficial medicine to official medicine. Perhaps ironically, that commonality was what led to increasing official interference in the ecosystem of unofficial medical practice. Medical drugs were vital to early modern Russian medicine. Knowing this, we can explore these vital yet lost objects through the texts about them that have survived, beginning with the most common group: botanicals.

2

Muscovy's Botanical World

The Apothecary Chancery oaths and investigations tell us that when Muscovites were concerned with medicine, they were concerned with medical drugs. Examining the other sources of early modern Russian medical history, we find that one category of medical drugs was particularly common: plant-based drugs. Official and unofficial texts, books, and prescriptions, are all full of plants of various kinds. Medical books that circulated in early modern Russia did include other objects in their pages, but plants, flowers, herbs, and trees always took centre stage. The Apothecary Chancery employed an entire group of people, the *travniki*, whose job was to collect plants for use in medicines. Plants were important enough to the Apothecary Chancery that they had more than one apothecary garden, where they could grow certain plants as well as having them collected and imported. Just as early modern Russian medicine was dominated by a concern for medical drugs, the category of medical drugs was dominated by plant-based medicines.

This enthusiasm for botanicals led to an interest in global medicines. As early as the sixteenth century, Russians could read about and use natural objects from North Africa such as Alexandrine senna, South East Asia–like nutmeg, South Asia–like sandalwood, and East Asia–like rhubarb. Around 1600, this geography shifted. The department then also began importing an increasing quantity and variety of botanicals from the Americas, alongside a continued use of local and Afro-Eurasian plants. Both groups of plants were in regular use across the seventeenth and into the eighteenth centuries. This shift towards including American botanical medicines is significant: no other American product would be in regular and officially sanctioned use in Russia until the 1690s, when the tobacco ban instituted in 1628 was finally lifted. Russia's interest in botanicals became a de facto enthusiasm for the most global of medicines available in early modern Eurasia.

Such keenness for global botanicals is not a given. Some data, such as the London port books, indicate a robust interest in American botanicals in early modern Europe.[1] Yet in England not everyone with access to the American botanicals approved of them. Alix Cooper has written about certain British authors "inventing the indigenous," turning away from foreign ingredients like the American botanicals and instead relying heavily on local ingredients.[2] In contrast, in Russia there was a growing quantity and variety of American drugs in official use, always employed in conjunction with local ingredients. Many medical cultures had access to foreign ingredients; not all of them chose to use them. The presence of American ingredients in Muscovy is significant because it shows approval of that kind of ingredient.

Russian use of American plants takes us back to considerations of timing and global change. Columbus first invaded the Americas in 1492. The Spanish physician Nicolás Bautista Monardes published on American medical botany in 1571. American drugs start appearing in Russian records in the 1600s. There was then a lag between the first European incursions into the Americas and the uptake of American drugs in Western Europe, and another gap between the uptake of American drugs in Western Europe and their first mentions in Russian documents. Heng provides a way of thinking about this as an "asynchrony of global temporalities," connections between regions forming or dissolving at different times.[3] Russia's connection to the Americas formed at a different time from Spain's connection, and did so for important reasons. Columbus did not know about which American drugs were going to be valuable in 1492. In the 1570s Monardes was promoting some of those drugs as valuable, but this was part of a process of convincing Eurasians of the benefit of buying new goods the supply of which was then controlled by the Spanish Empire. Russians begin purchasing and using American drugs when their value had been established in Afro-Eurasia. The activities of people like Columbus and Monardes made that decision possible, but it was the Russian enthusiasm for botanicals regardless of origin that made it happen.

TRANSLATING THE GARDEN

On 4 May 1534, a group of men sat in a room in Novgorod, the ancient East Slavic city and long-time trading partner of Western European merchants, to finish translating a book. One man was Nicolaus Bülow, a physician from the northern German Hansestadt of Lübeck, once again serving as medical practitioner to a Russian dignitary. He had spent much of his career travelling from his hometown to his not-quite-adopted nation, acting as medic, adviser, and sometime translator.[4] He was joined by a Russian translator, who collaborated with Bülow in rendering the book from low German into Church Slavonic. They may have been joined on this day by the man who had commissioned the translation, Metropolitan Daniil, a church leader based in Moscow. It was the scriptorium of Daniil's Metropolitan residence in which they all sat, surrounded by other copyists working on everything from encyclopedias to the Bible, and all surrounded by reams upon reams of paper.[5] Daniil was a major figure in sixteenth-century Russia. A disciple of the great Russian abbot Iosif Volotskii, he was for a time hegumen of the monastery bearing Iosif's name, before becoming Metropolitan and deeply involved with the politics of Grand Prince Vasilii III, sanctioning the divorce that ended Vasilii's childless first marriage to Solomonia Saburova.[6]

Yet even the presence of a giant of his times like Daniil was not the most important part of this scene. More important than the men was the *book*. The work being translated was the *Garden of Health*, an herbal enumerating plants and other natural objects and their medical uses, compiled by Johan von Kube as the *Gaerde der Sundheit* in 1485, and reprinted multiple times, including in Bülow's Lübeck in 1492. Bülow's copy of the 1492 text was with them, serving as the basis of their translation, the *Blagoprokhladnyi vertograd*. From its origins in the Novgorod scriptorium, this manuscript was sent to the Moscow Kremlin, political, spiritual, and medical centre of the empire, and passed through many hands before landing, much, much, later in a more southerly city.[7] This first translation spawned a multitude of other Slavonic texts of the *Garden of Health*, with major new copies being created in 1616 and 1672. In fact, the *Garden of Health* was the most copied medical text of early modern Russia, making up perhaps half the number of known Russian-language medical books from the seventeenth and eighteenth centuries, with a handful of nineteenth-century copies to boot.[8] These texts, like all Russian-language medical books before the 1730s, circulated exclusively in manuscript; the Slavonic *Garden of Health* was never printed.[9] These works were owned by the Apothecary Building and its successors, but also by tsars and nobles, monks and merchants. If one wanted to read only one source on early modern Russian medicine, it would be this book.

The first translation of the *Garden of Health*, completed in that paper-filled room in Novgorod in the summer of 1534, has understandably attracted much attention, and, equally understandably, much frustration. For a long time, a large part of the frustration was caused by the absence of the manuscript itself, thought lost, as were so many other sixteenth-century works. But in 2001, a manuscript held by Kharkiv national university library was identified by B.N. Morozov as the 1534 *Garden of Health*.[10] Since that first bold claim, a number of scholars have put forward their views on the security of this identification, on the relationship of other major *Garden of Health* manuscripts to the 1534 text and to each other, as well as on the ownership and history of these manuscripts.[11] Yet one notable aspect has yet to receive much attention: the 1534 *Garden of Health* as a medical work. Despite all the scrutiny the manuscript has received, almost nothing has been said about the point of this text: the kind of medicine it contains. Here, then, of all the points we may or may not have established about the 1534 text, we will focus on the least studied and most vital question for the history of medicine in early modern Russia: the kinds of drugs it recommends.

Presuming, as most scholars presently do, that the Kharkiv manuscript is either the 1534 text or a later sixteenth-century creation, we can use this text as our starting point for looking at plants in herbals.[12] The Kharkiv manuscript contains 688 chapters, each devoted to a natural object. Of the 688 chapters, the book itself describes 542 of those chapters as relating to *travy*, herbs, although a handful of these are not as herb-like as one might expect: milk, water, meat, bread, and cheese are all included in this section. Nevertheless, 530 of the chapters describe a plant. The other 146 chapters that the book does not list as "herbs" are devoted to stones or animals.[13] The Kharkiv manuscript, and thus likely the 1534 text, describes a variety of objects, but is dominated by one major category: plants.

We know rather more about the later Slavonic copies of the *Garden of Health* than we do about the 1534 text. The most important copy is that produced in 1616.[14] We have an origin story for this manuscript, too: the copyist, Flor, wrote an introduction to the herbal, in which he recounts a dramatic and romantic tale of returning to the Moscow Kremlin in 1612 following its sack by Polish forces, searching the ruins for surviving books, and finding this treasure house of medico-botanical knowledge. It is from Flor's manuscript that we gain much of the history of the *Garden of Health* for, alongside his own tale of discovering the text, he also provides much of the history of the 1534 translation. The 1616 manuscript is vital to understanding the *Garden of Health* in Russia.

From 1616 on, the Slavonic *Garden of Health* went through several changes. The 1616 text contains 687 chapters, of which 542 are devoted to plants and animals, the rest to minerals, and it has multiple additional sections.[15] The other major copy is the 1672 Filagrii manuscript, copied by Filagrii, the Patriarch's treasurer. This text changes the name of the work a little – from the *Blagoprokhladnyi vertograd*, it becomes the *Prokhladnyi vertograd* – and adds a number of sections, in particular religious texts relating to healing.[16] Despite a range of changes to the Slavonic *Garden of Health* as it was copied, recopied, and adapted across the seventeenth, eighteenth, and even into the nineteenth century, the majority of copies contain at least 500 chapters on plants, and around 140 on stones, minerals, and animal parts.[17] The *Garden of Health* changed in a variety of ways across the course of some three centuries – a new name, new sections, a changing selection of chapters – but the core of the text remained plants and their medicinal uses.

We can also trace the kinds of plants in the *Garden of Health*. Some of them were those that could be found locally, like the flower *chernobyl*, which the 1616 *Garden of Health* lists with a Latin and a Russian name, or kitchen-garden dill, similarly implying that it grew locally. Some were European plants more generally, like rosemary, or were given a name with a European origin point, like Polish dill or Venetian turpentine. Others came from farther afield. The term used for senna in this text, *Aleksandreiskii list*, implies a connection with Alexandrine senna, and so with North Africa where that plant grows. Others have origin-point names from farther East, such as Persian Apple, or Indian leaf. Still others are known to have grown in specific regions, like nutmeg from the Maluku Islands in Southeast Asia, or rhubarb, the best early modern varieties of which were grown in China (the near-ubiquitousness of rhubarb in modern Europe is the result of a long history of experiments by early modern botanists to get the most desirable variety of this plant to grow in

Europe).[18] In short, the plants listed in the Slavonic *Garden of Health* were not exclusively from the Russian Empire, nor from Europe, but derived from a wide range of places across Afro-Eurasia.[19]

The Slavonic *Garden of Health* manuscript was one of several herbals circulating in sixteenth-century Russia. The 1492 low German *Garden of Health* seems to have been kept in the Moscow Kremlin.[20] A late sixteenth-century library list contains one herbal from the Apothecary Building that Tsar Ivan IV kept in his bedchamber.[21] Medical texts also circulated outside of the walls of the Kremlin. Several notable families and figures, including the merchant family the Stroganovs, the noble I.P. Cheliadin, and the military governor [*voevoda*] I.M. Buturlin, owned herbals, although little is known about those texts.[22] Significantly, other than herbals the vast majority of other texts circulating in sixteenth-century Muscovy were religious texts.[23] Literacy was not a valued noble habit in sixteenth-century Muscovy, and the Russian elite owned fewer books than their Western European contemporaries. The existence of multiple herbals like the *Garden of Health* within the Kremlin then indicates that this was a genre of substantial value to the Russian elite.

The Slavonic *Gardens of Health* are the most important of a major genre of texts circulating early modern Russia, the herbal. Despite a general disinterest in reading among the sixteenth-century Russian elite, herbals were owned by many key figures, demonstrating the value that Muscovites placed on them. Based on surviving manuscripts, we can see what kinds of *materia medica* these texts recommended to their Muscovite owners. First and foremost, they recommended plants above all other kinds of natural objects. Even more important is the geographical origin of the plants recommended in these texts. This includes plants that grew within the Russian Empire, and Russia's trading partners in Western Europe, but also in Asia and Africa. The *materia medica* recommended by the Slavonic *Gardens of Health* to its Muscovite readers was an Afro-Eurasian botanical world.

PRESCRIBING THE GARDEN

The 1534 *Garden of Health*, with its wealth of knowledge about herbs from across the Old World, was often kept with other works offering similar insights into the medicinal properties of the natural world. Although the 1534 *Garden of Health* began its life in the Novgorod scriptorium, it did not stay there for long, and by the second half of the sixteenth century it was in the Moscow Kremlin, most likely in the library of the Apothecary Building [*Aptechnaia izba*].[24] In that library, it would have been kept in a box or a chest, a large storage case meant to protect manuscripts, the valuable work of many months. The Apothecary Building library boxes contained other similar works.[25] The purpose of these texts was related to the purpose of the department: to create medical drugs. Of the very few fragments of evidence relating to the department in the late sixteenth century, there are eight surviving prescriptions from 1581–82. Those prescriptions allow us to compare the theory of medical drugs contained in texts like the *Garden of Health* to the reality of practice in the department.

The survival story of the 1580s prescriptions provides a prosaic counterpoint to the romantic tale of Flor coming across the 1534 *Garden of Health* as he scoured the ransacked Kremlin for surviving manuscripts. The prescriptions were rediscovered in the Military Chancery [*Razriad*] files, as they had been used as *oblozhniki* [covers] for other, more important, documents.[26] The 1534 *Garden of Health* survived as a hidden treasure in an occupied stronghold; the 1580s prescriptions survived as scrap paper. Despite their rather grubby survival story, the 1580s prescriptions are treasures for historians of medicine.

Prescriptions as a genre of medical text are rather rare survivals. These often small, scrappy documents were medical ephemera, designed to hold a list of ingredients, the name of the compound being created, perhaps the recipe itself, often the name of the physician and the apothecary involved, even the name of the patient. In Western Europe, they were commonly written by the physician, a member of the medical group responsible for deciding the course of treatment, and given to the apothecary, the practitioner responsible for sourcing, stocking, and creating medicines. In the Russian case, the prescriptions reveal that they were written by a small group of Western European physicians then in service to the court and made up by Western European apothecaries under the orders of both the doctors and the head of department, Arms-Bearer [*oruzhnichii*] B.Ia. Bel'skii.

The 1580s prescriptions also mention some patients, high-level members of court, but, notably, not the tsar or his family, and not all the prescriptions include the name of the patient. There are two possible explanations for these gaps. First, as suggested by G.V. Zharinov, prescriptions given to Bel'skii may have been destined for the tsar – using the Apothecary Building director as a medical courier for the tsar was standard practice in the seventeenth century.[27] Alternatively, prescriptions for the tsar may have been stored separately, as was also standard practice in the seventeenth century. Documents relating to the tsar's health were always treated with more care than other Apothecary Building documents, so it is also plausible that only the records of less important patients were recycled as *oblozhniki*, and the tsar's prescriptions were stored, and lost, in a different fashion. These treasures of medical history, then, are hugely valuable, and fundamentally incomplete, meaning they must be used, but with caution.

The eight surviving prescriptions thus allow an all-too-rare glimpse into medical practices at the sixteenth-century Russian court. We can see these processes more clearly by examining one such recipe:

> The year 7090 [1581], November the 15th day. According to [the order of] Ivan Iakovlevich Bel'skii, Doctor Ivan [was permitted] to take [the following to make a prescription]: 3 *zolotniki*[28] of Alexandrine senna, 4 *zolotniki* of athamanta turbith, 2 *zolotniki* of Indian myrobalan plum,[29] 2 and a half *zolotniki* of rhubarb, a *zolotnik* each of anise and saffron.[30]

One point that emerges from this text is the geography of the *materia medica* being used. Senna alexandrina grew in several places around North Africa and the Middle East but was most closely associated with the present-day regions of Egypt and Sudan. Athamanta turbith, anise, and saffron all grow around the Mediterranean. The myrobalan plum is here specifically identified as being from India. Early modern rhubarb, especially that present in Russia, came from China.

The recipe from 15 November 1581 is representative of the 1580s prescriptions as a whole. It contains six ingredients, all of which are plant-based. The shortest prescription contains just two ingredients and the longest fifty-nine, with the median number being nine. There are 112 ingredients listed in all the 1580s prescriptions, with eighty-one, or around 70 per cent, being identifiable (see Appendix One for the full list). Of the identified items, all but one are plant-based; the exception is *tera sizilata*, terra sigillata, a kind of medicinal earth. No known terms for chemical or flesh-based medicines are included in these prescriptions. The *materia medica* listed in the 1580s prescriptions, just like the *materia medica* included in the Slavonic *Garden of Health*, are overwhelmingly plant-based.

The geographical origin of the materials listed in the 1580s prescriptions as a whole is also significant. One ingredient was specific to the Russian Empire: Don poppies, a reference to the Southern river that flows into the Sea of Azov. One ingredient was specific to Europe: *renskoe vino*, Rhenish wine, from the German-speaking wine region of Rheinhessen. Several others could have been sourced from multiple possible locations: mint and juniper berries both grow in various places. Particularly notable is the presence of materials associated with Africa and Asia. As well as the North African senna alexandrina, there is also West African gum Arabic. Asia provided galangal, ginger, saffron, cardamom, cinnamon. The Maluku Islands (Moluccas), known to early modern Europeans as the Spice Islands, provided cloves and nutmeg. [31] No known terms for American products are included in these documents. Again, like the Slavonic *Garden of Health*, the 1580s prescriptions include materials from around Afro-Eurasia but not the Americas.

If we look more closely at the contents of the 1580s prescriptions and the Slavonic *Garden of Health*, the issue of similarity becomes more complicated. The 1580s prescriptions list 110 different ingredients.[32] The Kharkiv manuscript of the Slavonic *Garden of Health* contains 688 chapters, 542 of them relating to herbs.[33] In other words, even if the contents of these two sets of documents perfectly lined up, the 1580s prescriptions would include less than 20 per cent of the contents of the *Garden of Health*. However, the 1580s prescriptions and the *Garden of Health* do not perfectly line up. Let us take the prescription from 15 November 1581 as an example. The *Garden of Health* does have specific chapters on Athamanta turbith, rhubarb, and anise, yet the *Garden of Health* does not provide the specific recipes created in the 1580s. Rather, it provides general medico-botanical information about the natural objects it lists.[34] If the *Garden of Health* was one of the reference texts consulted in creating these prescriptions, it would have provided only a part of the picture. The Slavonic *Garden of Health* would have been a helpful resource in creating the prescriptions of the 1580s because the two sets of documents share a common view on medicaments, but they do not completely overlap.

Considering the process of creating these prescriptions, which brought together plants from across the known world by way of Moscow's service staff and equipment, also brings us to the language problem. The medical staff of the Apothecary Building in the 1580s were mostly English and German, and they knew Latin but not Slavic languages. The bureaucratic staff were exclusively Russian. The Slavonic *Garden of Health* is in Church Slavonic. It is in Russian that these prescriptions survive, although, if seventeenth-century standard practice was followed in the 1580s, then these are translations from Latin drafts.[35] In order for the apothecaries to create these prescriptions, the Apothecary Building staff had to catalogue, store, and retrieve all the ingredients. There were translators, but those translators had no specific training in medical affairs. The prescriptions themselves do not tell us how this language situation was navigated.

Medical practitioners at the court themselves seem to have been concerned over the language issue. The earliest existing Russian-English dictionary is attributed to Mark Ridley, an English physician who worked at the court in 1594–99.[36] The dictionary lists a number of medical terms, and also includes what Ridley termed "classified vocabularies," what we might alternatively call word lists: one of these lists is of plants. Notably, the list of plants is by far the longest, with nearly four times as many items as the classified vocabulary of diseases.[37] Ridley's list bears an interesting relationship to both the 1580s prescriptions and the *Garden of Health*. Only half the ingredients of the 1581 recipe quoted above can be clearly identified in Ridley's text: rhubarb, anise, and saffron.[38] Ridley's dictionary would have been helpful to a physician engaged with the plant-focused Afro-Eurasian *materia medica* of late sixteenth-century official Russian medicine, but, like the Slavonic *Garden of Health*, it did not provide a complete guide to that world.

Expanding our view of sixteenth-century official Russian medicine beyond the *Garden of Health* and into the practice of prescribing shows us some issues in understanding this world, but also underlines one major fact about it. The fragments of sixteenth-century official medicine that have survived – the Kharkiv manuscript, the Ridley dictionary, and the 1580s prescriptions – give only a partial view of what happened in the Apothecary Building. Yet they are united in two key ways. All the extant documents focus on plants as *materia medica*, to the near-total exclusion of all other objects. Those plants came from across Afro-Eurasia, both from regions with which the Russian court had close ties and regions with which they did not. We cannot answer all questions about the creation of medical drugs at the sixteenth-century Russian court, but we can show that it was Old World plants, above all other objects, that were prized as ingredients for medicines.

THE OLD BOTANICAL WORLD

The medico-botanical world view exemplified by the *Garden of Health* was long-lived within the Russian Empire. We can trace certain specific commodities, and through them, the more general appreciation of Afro-Eurasian botanical medicaments from the 1530s to the 1750s. Such tracking can be tricky. Afro-Eurasian botanicals were widely traded and used in medicine for centuries, and this often went hand in hand with botanical transfers, moving plants to new regions of cultivation. Tracking botanicals across the Old World is thus difficult, but careful selection of specific commodities demonstrates substantial continuity in the use of these products across the sixteenth, seventeenth, and eighteenth centuries.

Moving from the sixteenth century in to the seventeenth and eighteenth, we leave behind the fragmented traces of the Apothecary Building and encounter new institutions. The overwhelming majority of documents on early modern Russian medicine come from the Apothecary Chancery [*Aptekarskii prikaz*], which has left us a wide range of files, including a substantial collection of prescriptions, import lists, and stocktaking documents. Looking at the eighteenth century, we come across the extensive files of the Apothecary Chancery's replacement, the Medical Chancellery [*Meditsinskaia kantsliariia*]. The records of eighteenth-century official Russian medicine are in some ways more extensive than those of the seventeenth century: these records take up 150 huge bound volumes to cover only the material from 1736 (when extant records begin) to 1750. These volumes include numerous detailed lists of what that department was sending to the Russian army, and multiple inventories, but no prescriptions to individuals.[39] The records of the Apothecary Chancery and the Medical Chancellery allow us to continue to track plant-based *materia medica* used at court in the 1580s into the seventeenth and eighteenth centuries.

Returning to our recipe of 1581 that we examined above, one particular commodity is significant: rhubarb.[40] The Russian Empire had been aware of rhubarb and its medicinal applications, particularly as a diuretic, from at least the sixteenth century. Like Western Europe, Russians valued a particular variety of rhubarb commonly sourced from China and set up a state monopoly on the trade in that rhubarb within the empire, a trade facilitated by Bukharan merchants, who brought the plant to Russian trading posts.[41] Erika Monahan has shown that there was a short-lived attempt to source the valued kind of rhubarb within the Russian Empire, but it was quickly abandoned.[42] When we find rhubarb in early modern Russian medical documents, we are finding an East Asian product.

The prescriptions of the Apothecary Chancery show rhubarb in regular use. It was commonly prescribed to high-ranking court figures, such as Tsar Mikhail Fedorovich and the Danish Count Valdemar in 1645.[43] That use of rhubarb at court continued across the seventeenth century, as it is listed in prescriptions from the 1660s to the 1690s.[44] It was also among the supplies the department sent to the Russian army, seen on a list of materials from 1662.[45] Looking at the records of the Medical Chancellery, we see that they had rhubarb in stock from the 1730s to at least the 1750s.[46] East Asian rhubarb, valued by the Russian Empire as a major resale commodity for transport to the West, was also commonly used within official Russian medicine from the late sixteenth to the mid-eighteenth century.

Along with rhubarb, the 1581 recipe also lists Senna alexandrina, a commodity with a North African association.[47] Links between the Russian Empire and Africa are not commonly discussed: various works have been published on Russia's trade with both Western Europe and East Asia, but African links have not been given the same attention.[48] François-Xavier Fauvelle has emphasised the extensive pre-modern trade connections of various African polities and cities, although he does not specifically mention links with the East Slavic lands.[49] Nevertheless, such links did exist. In the ninth and tenth centuries, the Volga Bulgars, whose lands would later be conquered by the Russian Empire, were trading Siberian furs to, among other places, North Africa.[50] At least by the 1690s, Russia imported enslaved Africans.[51] The importation of North African senna was one way in which North Africa and the Russian Empire were linked by trade and commodities.

Like rhubarb, we also commonly find senna in seventeenth- and eighteenth-century Russian prescriptions, and indeed sometimes in the same places. When Tsar Mikhail Fedorovich and the Danish Count Valdemar received rhubarb in 1645, they also received senna.[52] Top Apothecary Chancery doctor Laurentius Blumentrost prescribed it in 1672.[53] It was sent to the army in 1648 and 1663.[54] The Medical Chancellery here again followed the example of the Apothecary Chancery, keeping senna in stock across the early eighteenth century.[55] Africa, the extent of whose links with the premodern Russian Empire remain largely unexplored, certainly provided them with senna across the sixteenth, seventeenth, and eighteenth centuries.

Another piece of specific botanical geography is provided by what were once called by Europeans the Spice Islands, the Maluku Islands. The Maluku Islands were long the sole growing region of a number of highly valued botanical commodities, including the products of the Myristica tree, mace and nutmeg. When we find nutmeg and mace anywhere in the pre-modern world, we know they came from the Maluku Islands. Nutmeg was used in official Russian medicine, being found in the 1580s prescriptions, the seventeenth-century import lists of the Apothecary Chancery, and in numerous Apothecary Chancery prescriptions, including a collection from the 1660s.[56] The Medical Chancellery also had it in stock in the 1730s.[57] The official prescriptions of the Russian Empire show the continuous presence of botanicals specific to Southeast Asia from the 1580s to the mid-eighteenth century.

The routes by which these botanicals reached Russia were several and were determined by diplomacy, colonialism, and trading links rather than geographical logic. A major source of African and Asian commodities for the Russian court was Western Europe, notably their major diplomatic and trade contacts, the Netherlands, the German lands, and England.[58] This route, which meant Asian commodities were shipped west via the southern coast of Africa, was a very long one, created by European colonialism in Asia and Africa and the diplomatic and trading patterns of Europe. Some Asian commodities did take the land route to Moscow, notably rhubarb.[59] We know Armenian, Bukharan, and Indian merchants all played a role in importing other Asian commodities to Russia across Eurasia, including medicinal commodities.[60] The routes along which senna, rhubarb, and nutmeg were traded were always long, but sometimes even longer than we might have supposed, as European colonialism warped global trade routes around itself.

In addition to the importation of botanicals from across Afro-Eurasia, prescriptions also tell us something about the internal medical botanical activities of the Russian Empire. Both Kirill Khudin and Rachel Koroloff have written about the *travniki*, the herb collectors of the empire, who were officially tasked with gathering a range of plants for use by the

Apothecary Chancery, such as juniper berries.[61] The department prescribed those berries several times across the seventeenth century.[62] The Medical Chancellery also kept them in stock and sent some to the army in the 1730s and 1750s.[63] As well as their substantial use of foreign connections, the departments of official Russian medicine made use of local resources across the seventeenth and eighteenth centuries.

This use of local botanicals also tells us something more about connections between official and unofficial medicine in Russia. A.B. Ippolitova has worked on Russian ethnobotany, showing the common use of plants, and local plants in particular, in early modern unofficial medicine. Also importantly, Ippolitova's work has shown substantial long-term continuity in the use of the unofficial medical texts she studies, with some being used or copied from the seventeenth to the twentieth centuries.[64] In healing-related witchcraft trials, the physical evidence presented was invariably a plant of some kind.[65] Unofficial Russian medicine of the seventeenth century agreed with official Russian medicine on the general value of plant-based medicines, and on the specific value of local plants in those medicines.

The records of the Apothecary Chancery and the Medical Chancellery, as well as the more scattered records of unofficial Russian medicine, allow us to track the interests of Muscovites in plant-based medicines into the seventeenth and eighteenth centuries. Both unofficial and official medicine in this period maintained a focus on plant-based medicines and used plants local to the Russian Empire. The official departments, with their international connections through the court, were able and willing to import plant medicines from elsewhere. We already know much about the international trading connections of Muscovy with Western Europe; looking at medical documents shows us that there was a long-term importation and use of plants from East and Southeast Asia, and Africa across this period. The enthusiasm for Afro-Eurasian plant-based medicines that we saw in the *Garden of Health* and the 1580s prescriptions continued for over a century.

THE FOURTH PART OF THE WORLD

Official Russian medicine made substantial use of plants from across Afro-Eurasia from the 1580s on. There is one other major origin point of plant medicines used in Afro-Eurasia in this period: the Americas. From the sixteenth century on, an increasing number of medicinal plants were imported from European colonies in the Americas and taken up by medical practitioners and sufferers across Afro-Eurasia. The immediate issue with investigating the Russian Empire's level of knowledge and use of American medicaments is that the beginning of Russian involvement in the Americas is typically dated to 1732, when an Academy of Sciences expedition sighted the Aleutian Islands. This event kicked off a creeping colonization of the region by the Russian Empire, ending in 1867 when the colony of Russian America was sold to the United States and became Alaska.[66] Little work has thus far been devoted to Russian knowledge of the Americas before 1732. In order to understand the Russian Empire's knowledge and use of American plant drugs, we first need to know their overall level of involvement in, and knowledge of, Eurasian-American interactions before 1732.

When we look at existing histories of trade and commodities, there is little evidence of American goods coming to Russia before the eighteenth century. Jarmo Kotilaine's work on Russia's foreign trade in the seventeenth century makes no mention of any American goods coming to Russia in that period.[67] Potatoes were supposedly first brought to Russia by Tsar Peter the Great in 1716, but were unpopular until the nineteenth century.[68] V.N. Zakharov found little indication of imports from the Americas even as late as the mid-eighteenth century.[69] Matthew P. Romaniello has shown that tobacco was known in the Russian Empire in the seventeenth century, but it was banned between 1628 and 1697, making this more an example of a lack of connection.[70] Looking at the established histories of trade and commodities, there is little trace of exchanges between the Americas and Russia before the eighteenth century.

Looking at texts gives us a different perspective. A document from the early sixteenth century is key to the history of Russian-American relations. Around 1530 Maxim Grek, a Greek monk who worked for the Russian court in the late fifteenth and early sixteenth centuries, wrote:

> And Ancient people did not know, or did not want, to travel through Gadir; modern Spanish and Portuguese people, sailing in great ships with much danger, have recently – 40 or 50 years ago, at the end of the seventh millennium[71] – [done so] and found many islands, some empty, and a great land called Cuba, the extent of which is not known by those who live there. Finding this, they travelled around

> the whole southern land, even to the East of the Winter Sun, to India, to the seven islands known as the Maluku Islands,[72] in which grow cinnamon and cloves and other fragrant aromatics, which until now were not known to a single human, and now are all known to the king of the Spanish and the Portuguese.[73]

The geography here is varied and perplexing. We have references to Spain and Portugal (including the port of Gadir, an old name for Cadiz), Cuba, India, and the Maluku Islands. To understand which voyage Grek is describing, we need to unpack this text.

There are two vital clues as to which voyage this is. First of all, the date. Grek was writing ca 1530 and notes that the voyage took place forty to fifty years earlier, which puts the voyage he describes in the 1480s or 1490s. The second clue is the repeated reference to this voyage as something new. Ancient people did not make this journey, and those modern people who did discovered islands previously unseen by Europeans, we are told, indicating that this is an entirely new route, such as that found by Columbus in 1492. When the text moves to describing the botanical wonders acquired on the journey, it mentions that along the route the voyagers came across botanicals not previously known to Europeans, as American commodities were not in the 1490s. The text also references Cuba, which Columbus visited, and Cádiz, from which Columbus departed on some of his American voyages in the 1490s. These elements of the text then look very much like a description of Columbus's early voyages to the Caribbean in the 1490s, a conclusion that major historians of Russian America like N.N. Bolkhovitinov have made.[74]

Yet there are other elements in this passage that fit less well with Columbus's voyages. The references to rounding a Southern land, to India, the Maluku Islands, and to Asian commodities like cinnamon and cloves, have no place in a retelling of the Columbus voyages. Those parts of the text more closely resemble Ferdinand Magellan's 1519 voyage around the southern coast of South America, ending up in the Maluku Islands, where cloves originate. But, as with the Columbus voyage, this interpretation does not entirely fit the text. Magellan did not depart from Cádiz, did not visit Cuba, and his voyage did not take place forty to fifty years prior to 1530. Here it is important to remember that the European understandings of the geography of the Americas, and their relationship to Asia, were evolving over the sixteenth century, and that textual transmission across

Europe and between different languages often led to texts changing significantly or becoming confused. One reading of the Grek text is that it conflates the Columbus and Magellan voyages, creating an account of a hybrid Spanish-sponsored voyage to the Americas. The earliest known text on the Americas available to the Russian court then presents a rather confused picture of the European invasions but, significantly for our purposes, linked that geography to valuable botanical commodities.

Following Grek's 1530 account, the Americas then appeared in a number of sixteenth- and seventeenth-century Russian documents. There was a letter on Magellan's voyages, as well as the translation of Martyn Bielskii's *Chronicle of the Whole World* [*Khronika vsego sveta*] in which the Americas are called the "fourth part of the world."[75] The Ambassadorial Chancery [*Posol'skii prikaz*], responsible for Muscovy's foreign relations, created several texts relating to the Americas. Some were stand-alone reports, such as Andrei Vinius's on the colony of New Spain.[76] Others were part of a series: the *Vesti-Kuranty*, translations of selected excerpts of Western European newspapers that highlighted the news most of interest to the tsar and his advisers, repeatedly mention the Americas and more specifically European actions in the Americas.[77] From the 1530s to the 1690s, the Russian elite could learn about the Americas, and in particular European activities there, from a range of texts then available to them.

The textual presence of the Americas in documents like the *Vesti-Kuranty* was joined, by the end of the seventeenth century, by visual depictions of the Americas. Between 1697 and 1711 the famous Siberian cartographer Semyon Remezov produced his "Chronographic Sketchbook," a collection of maps. In his conclusion to this work, Remezov also directly references the Americas, calling his work an atlas "of the entire interior of Siberia, with the reigning city of Tobolsk and the cities, settlements, forts and parishes under its jurisdiction, especially between the countries [*sic*] of Asia, Europe and America."[78] In the same work, he also reproduced a Dutch two-hemisphere world map that includes the Americas.[79] Following sixteenth- and earlier seventeenth-century Russian documents that copied Western European texts about the Americas, by the 1690s Russian documents were also reproducing Western European images of the Americas.

The currently known history of pre-1700 Russian-American interactions is mixed. Major commodities were either not introduced until later, like the potato, or were banned, like tobacco. Texts were written about the Americas from the early sixteenth century on, but some of them present a confused view of the geography of the region and the events taking place during the European invasions of the Americas. Visual depictions of the Americas seem to have been produced only at the very end of the seventeenth century. Despite this idiosyncratic view of pre-1700 Russian–American interactions, the Russian elite were aware of the Americas and of the presence there of valuable commodities. We can now turn to the question of whether they directly experienced American commodities in their medicines.

EVERYDAY AMERICANA

The Russian elite knew about the Americas at least as early as the 1530s, yet extant prescriptions from the 1580s show no American ingredients, nor does the *Garden of Health* include any. A century later, Apothecary Chancery records mentioned several such plants. From at least 1602, and more intensively from the 1660s, official Russian medicine imported, processed, stored, and prescribed American plant medicines harvested from multiple locations across the two continents. These medicinal objects were originally the property of the Indigenous peoples of the Americas, as all Eurasian knowledge of the properties of American plants was fundamentally derived from Indigenous experts but were primarily brought to Russia by Western European middlemen.[80] Sixteenth-century Russian medicine was global, in the sense that it used ingredients from around Afro-Eurasia. Seventeenth-century Russian medicine was globalized, in the sense that it continued to use Afro-Eurasian ingredients but now in combination with American botanicals. Russian enthusiasm for plant-based medicines led to a globalization of medical ingredients, in particular from the late sixteenth into the seventeenth century.

American medicaments were prescribed by the Apothecary Chancery to their elite patients, giving us particular detail regarding their use. During his final illness in 1645, Tsar Mikhail Fedorovich was prescribed an American medicament as a part of a series of recipes. On 24 April 1645, the Apothecary Chancery made up the following recipe for him:

> *Roots:* Althaea officinalis 6 *zolotniki.* Chicory, Scorzonera, *Polypodium,* Parsley, *Ononidis* of any kind, 3 *zolotniki* [each]. Inula, Orris, 2 *zolotniki* [each]. Capparis root bark[81] 6 *zolotniki.*

Herbs: Veronica, Agrimonia, Camedris of any kind, a handful [of each]. Woodworm 2 pinches.
Flowers: Rose, viola, 2 pinches [of each]. Primula veris, laserpitium siler, a pinch [of each]. Akikhenki berries[82], 3 *zolotniki*. Sassafras wood 3 *zolotniki*. Cinnamon 3 *zolotniki*. Cloves[83] 2 and a half *zolotniki*. Ginger 2 *zolotniki*. Alexandrine senna 12 *zolotniki*. Black Michoacán, Rhubarb 3 *zolotniki* [each]. Gelebri nigri[84] root half a *zolotnik*. Amelanchier berries 12 *zolotniki*. Cream of Tartar 2 *zolotniki*. A pinch of Rosemary. Aniseed 3 *zolotniki*. Juniper berries 6 *zolotniki*.
Rhenish wine mixed with various herbs and roots.[85]

This one long recipe can tell us several things, not only about the treatment of the tsar on this specific day, but about prescriptions of this period more generally.

In part, this recipe demonstrates the difficulties of identifying and translating historical Slavic botanical terms. Plants that share their Russian name with another European language – like Veronica – or those used in other contexts – for example, spices like cinnamon – can be quickly and fairly confidently identified. Others prove trickier. *Gvozdika* can mean either cloves or carnations; here the former seems more probable a translation, but that does not mean that this word in this document definitely means cloves, as flowers were a common part of early modern medicine. Other terms are entirely obscure. With the exception of Ridley's *Dictionary of the Vulgar Russe Tongue*, contemporary and historical dictionaries spend very little time on plants; botanical dictionaries by N. Annenkov and L.A. Utkin provide some help, but are focused on modern usage.[86] On the occasions that the historical dictionaries do list a plant name, they often lead in a frustrating circle back to the very document we are trying to translate. This is an issue for various regions: László Károly's edition of one of the rare Chagatai Turkic medical texts, composed in Bukhara in the seventeenth century, contains a number of footnotes stating that certain items are yet to be identified.[87] We can identify and translate a proportion of early modern Russian botanical terms, which give vital insight into the extant traces of that medicine. But such translations are never perfect reconstructions of that medico-botanical world.

From the terms we can confidently identify, we can see the geographical origins of certain plants. In this one recipe, we have some ingredients that were likely sourced locally. Parsley and rosemary both could have been collected near Moscow, as could juniper berries.[88] The most obvious ingredient from Western Europe is Rhenish wine. Other ingredients would have been brought in from Asia: rhubarb from China; cloves from South East Asia. Once again we see the African senna alexandrina. Two ingredients mark a notable change since 1581: sassafras and michoacán. Sassafras here means product of a tree that grows on the eastern seaboard of North America.[89] According to Daniela Bleichmar, michoacán root is a name used by early modern Spanish authors like Monardes, probably for what is also called jalap, from Mesoamerica.[90] This single recipe then shows us a geographic shift from exclusive use of Afro-Eurasian materials in the late sixteenth century, to materials from more than one location in the Americas by the middle of the seventeenth.

Identifying sassafras and michoacán allows us to further investigate these American commodities. Little is known about how early modern Indigenous Americans used michoacán root, but Monardes lists it as a purgative.[91] More is known about sassafras. Sassafras is most likely a French word for a tree known under several Native American names. We know the most about the Timucua nation of present-day Florida and their approach to this tree: they called it pauame, made tea from its roots to treat fevers, and were one of the main Native American groups from whom French and later Spanish invaders of the region learned of the tree and its medicinal properties. It would be the anti-febrile effects of sassafras, first discovered by the Timucua and other Native American groups, that Europeans would later rely upon in their use of the medicament. The Timucua and other Native American groups discovered the medicinal properties of sassafras, determined how to identify the tree, decided how to get the root, invented the anti-febrile tea, and were frequently responsible for harvesting that root for Europeans.[92] The indigenous medical botany of the Timucua and other Native American groups came to Moscow in the form of an object they in effect created.

The rest of the document to which this 1645 recipe belongs gives us an unusual level of detail regarding the reasons and theory of the treatment; this is the only recipe involving American medicaments for which we have an accompanying description of the proposed treatment. Before the beginning of the treatment, the tsar's doctors examined his urine, and declared the problem was that his "stomach and liver and spleen lack the natural warmth they need to create mucus. From this the blood is becoming somewhat thin, and [the patient] cold. This may lead to scurvy and other phlegmatic [lit. damp] illnesses."[93] This talk of natural heat and of cold, damp illnesses is typical of Galenic humoral medicine, where the aim was to balance the four humours of the body. Moreover, seventeenth-century medicine distinguished between "sea scurvy" and "land scurvy," with the latter considered a cold disease requiring hot remedies to counterbalance it.[94] By the eighteenth century, the environment of the vast Russian Empire, stereotyped as cold even then, was considered to commonly cause such land scurvy.[95] The presence of sassafras in particular here is then a little odd: it is best known as an antifebrile; following Galenic logic, it should then have been thought of as a cold herb and so inappropriate to treat Mikhail Fedorovich's lack of heat. The solution may be an issue of geography: both sassafras and michoacán root, from a continent stereotyped as hot, may have here been used as hot remedies for a cold disease. The remedies for Mikhail Fedorovich were Galenic, but the specific ingredients used do not entirely follow Galenic logic.

The sassafras and michoacán root given to Mikhail Fedorovich in 1645 were used throughout the seventeenth century. The earliest reference to an American plant in the Apothecary Chancery documents is to sassafras, in an import document from 1602; the earliest reference to the use of an American plant in the department is from 1633, when sassafras was sent to the army along with sarsaparilla, a blood purifier sourced from Brazil.[96] Sassafras in particular would be commonly used throughout the century: in a set of seventy-nine prescriptions from 1664–65, sassafras was prescribed nine times.[97] In the late seventeenth century, other American ingredients would appear in the prescriptions. By 1673, guaiacum, a South American plant most commonly used in Eurasia to treat syphilis, was being prescribed.[98] There was even one non-plant medicament: the Western Bezoar, most likely from the Andes, prescribed alongside the Eastern Bezoar the Muscovites had been using earlier.[99] Evidence from the 1680s is limited – only one small set of prescriptions survives from this period – but it shows continued use of American drugs, with sarsaparilla appearing in two of the five prescriptions.[100] This trend would continue into the 1690s, with sassafras, sarsaparilla, jalap, and guaiacum all in use.[101] In the late sixteenth century, there is no evidence of American medicaments being used in Russia; by the late seventeenth century, there were at least five such items in regular use.

Not only were there multiple American medicaments being consumed in Russia by the end of the century, they were often consumed in combination. For example, one Apothecary Chancery recipe from 25 December 1698 includes sarsaparilla, guaiacum, and sassafras, alongside china root, licorice, juniper berries, and aniseed.[102] Within one prescription we have three identifiable American medicaments combined with materials from elsewhere. It is also interesting to see sarsaparilla alongside china root [*radix Chinae*], as that Eastern plant was commonly considered the equivalent of sarsaparilla, with the latter sometimes called *radix China occidentalis*.[103] The recipe is half new world, half old world, with three American medicaments and four from Eurasia. The situation by the 1690s was for individual recipes to bring together multiple American ingredients with multiple Afro-Eurasian ingredients, integrating the American products into established *materia medica*.

In the eighteenth century, official medicine continued to use American medicines. Looking to the Medical Chancellery records shows that American drugs again come to the fore, with Peruvian balsam – produced from the bark of a South American tree similar to that from which cinchona bark was made, and with which it was often confused – being in stock in 1737.[104] Jalap was in stock in 1737 and 1738, as were sassafras and sarsaparilla from 1737.[105] Peruvian balsam appeared again in 1750, this time alongside the familiar guaiacum, sassafras, sarsaparilla, and jalap, as well as ipecacuanha, the root of the Brazilian cephaelis tree.[106] The Apothecary Chancery's enthusiasm for American *materia medica* was continued by the Medical Chancellery.

One notable imbalance appears in these records regarding the use of American plants in official Russian medicine: they were commonly prescribed to court figures, but much more rarely sent to the army.[107] It is possible that the reservation of certain goods for use by the court was due to price: one medicinal commodity exclusively restricted to the court was unicorn horn, one of the most expensive items per weight sold in early modern Europe.[108] Yet making calculations of the value of a medicament is tricky work. We have no extant document telling us the price per dose for each commodity, only some import documents listing bulk prices and some prescriptions listing quantities of items like sassafras by weight. Moreover, those prescriptions that do include quantities could differ by as much as twelve times the weight between prescriptions from the same year.[109] We cannot properly establish the specific monetary value of sassafras on the basis of such data. Rather, we do better to look at what sassafras and the other American botanicals represented. We know that there was a feeling in Eurasia that these were special commodities, a feeling that – judging by how both Maxim Grek and Samuel Collins wrote about them – was also present at the Russian court. Access to novel and exotic items is a form of status that one the rulers of Muscovy would have been unlikely to share with their soldiers. The American drugs, then, were primarily limited to courtly use as they were elite, even if they may not necessarily have been expensive.

We can also track American medicinal ingredients in Russia beyond the confines of the Apothecary Chancery and Medical Chancellery. In 1694, the Apothecary Chancery bought sassafras and cinchona from a Moscow market, meaning those two items were available to all customers of the market, official medical departments, unofficial medical practitioners, and sufferers alike.[110] In the early eighteenth century, the Russian government periodically revised tariffs on regularly traded goods, developments that Dutch merchants carefully tracked. In documents from 1724 and 1731 the Dutch record sassafras as an item with a standard tariff, meaning it was expected to be fairly regularly traded.[111] Jan Willem Veluwenkamp and Werner Scheltjens have shown that sarsaparilla was being imported into St Petersburg via the Danish Sound in the late eighteenth and into the nineteenth century.[112] In both cases, these imports were for sale on the open market, not supply runs for official departments. This data shows that there was at least some availability of American medicinal plants in the Russian Empire outside of official circles.

We also find some trace of American drugs in medical books aimed at a lay audience. There was a growing number of manuscript medical books being produced in Russian in the late seventeenth and into the eighteenth century. Many of them – including the *Pharmacopoeia for Domestic Use, Pharmacy for Transport and Service,* and the *Extract from Doctors' Knowledge* – do not mention any American drugs. Interestingly, the main text that does was produced for lay readers by an official department, the Academy of Sciences. *Florin's Economy,* a printed Russian translation of a German household work with multiple medical recipes, includes American drugs. Both sassafras and sarsaparilla are mentioned multiple times, often together, as in a recipe on weakness [*o rasslablenii*], included in both the 1738 and 1760 editions.[113] The evidence for American medical ingredients being used outside of official circles is limited, but it does exist.

The Russian Empire imported medical ingredients from an increasingly broad geography at great expense. We know in other contexts that such imports of expensive foreign ingredients either were opposed or an alternative was sought – for example, British Indian attempts to replace the American botanical cinchona with Swietenia febrifuga.[114] As discussed above, the Russian Empire did attempt to curtail their reliance on foreign rhubarb supplies, not by finding an alternative to rhubarb but rather by finding an alternative source of rhubarb within their territories, an attempt that ultimately failed.[115] The failed rhubarb experiment may point the way forward in understanding why the Russian Empire continued to use foreign goods such as nutmeg, senna, and sassafras. While local goods were cheaper, and easier to access and control, multiple goods were simply not available within the Empire at least until they began to be cultivated in the early eighteenth-century botanical and physic gardens.[116] The Russian Empire valued control of goods, but they also valued certain goods that grew only abroad, and were unwilling to replace those foreign goods, preferring, when possible, to instead source a foreign good locally.

In considering the Russian Empire's ongoing enthusiasm for materials as foreign as the American botanicals were, we can return here to Heng's point about "asynchrony of global temporalities," connections between regions forming or dissolving at different times.[117] Russia's connection to the Americas did not begin in 1492; rather, its textual relationship began in 1530, and its commodity exchange began in 1602. After that date, official Russian medicine in particular developed an interest in American medical ingredients that would last at least for the next century and a half. This new enthusiasm for American botanicals grew out of a prior interest in botanicals regardless of origin. Once the Russian elite was aware of the Americas, and once Western European middlemen had established the value of these new American plants, a new connection of official Russian medicine to Indigenous American herbal medicine was created. This was a globalization of Russian medicine, a widening of the geographical origin of its materials, that built on earlier global connections and took place on a schedule determined by the combination of the availability of the market and the interests of the Russian court.

CONCLUSION

Examining the materials of early modern Russian medicine reveals major aspects of that medical practice. Russia displayed a notable and consistent interest in plants as medical ingredients, an interest that we can see from the mid-sixteenth century through to the mid-eighteenth century. That interest in plants led to an increasingly global scope of Muscovite medicines. In the sixteenth century, the sources of Russian *materia medica* were already Afro-Eurasian; in contrast to the books and personnel of official Russian medicine that came from Western Europe, medical ingredients came from across the continent. This global focus was not automatic. Other medical practitioners in the early modern world valued specifically local plants; Russian medicine used local plants, but alongside foreign ones. The interest in plants was not based on origin, and so the enthusiasm for botanicals was initially an enthusiasm for Afro-Eurasian botanicals.

The 1600s saw a major shift in the geography of ingredients. This period saw the continued use of local and Afro-Eurasian plants, but it also saw the first importation and usage of American botanicals. Official Russian medicine in particular would then use an increasing range of American ingredients originating in different regions of the Americas throughout the seventeenth and into the eighteenth century. Those ingredients were considered valuable and trustworthy enough to be prescribed even to the tsar. This interest in medical drugs also took place in the near-total absence of any other American goods in pre-1700 Russia, showing a particular focus on medical ingredients. The interest in plant-based medicines globalized early modern Russian medicine, leading to a shift from Afro-Eurasian ingredients in the sixteenth century to Afro-Eurasian and American ingredients in the seventeenth and eighteenth. Following this most vital group of *materia medica,* we then see how a local enthusiasm for one category of objects led to a massive shift in the international connections of the Russian Empire.

3

Selling the Chemical Universe

From the sixteenth to the eighteenth centuries Russians had a particular enthusiasm for one kind of *materia medica*, plants. They were much more cautious about the use of other materials in medicines. One such material was chemicals. Putting chemicals in medicine, especially those chemicals known to be dangerous, was simultaneously common and controversial in the pre-modern world. There are pre-modern medical works from Tibet, South Asia, East Asia, and the Latin West that all recommend recipes including mercury; the latter, as in so many things, heavily relied upon earlier Arabic works.[1] In the Americas, pre-Columbian Aztec medical practitioners had their own chemical recipes.[2] By the middle of the sixteenth century, medical practitioners across the world had already been using chemical remedies for centuries.

Yet medical chemistry still managed to be new and revolutionary in early modern West Eurasia. Chemical medicine, also known as iatrochemistry or spagyric medicine, posed the earliest serious challenge to the centuries-old Galenic and Hippocratic dominance of European medical theory. Its key proponent was Paracelsus (born Philippus Aureolus Theophrastus Bombastus von Hohenheim, 1493–1541), a German-Swiss physician. His central idea concerned the balance of the three principles [*tria prima*] that made up the human body, which were represented by chemicals: salt was solidity or consistency, sulphur was inflammability or combustibility, and mercury was "spiritousness" or volatility. Paracelsus knew he was using materials known to be poisonous, including not only mercury but also arsenic.[3] Chemical medicine also revolutionized the production of medicines, promoting the extensive use of chemicals, and techniques such as distillation.[4] Paracelsus gave those century-old practices his own spin, and his works popularized them throughout Western Europe.

It was Paracelsian medicine, and its precipitous yet highly controversial rise in the late sixteenth and into the seventeenth century, that was significant to the Apothecary Chancery. First of interest in the German-speaking lands to which Paracelsus's German-language texts most directly appealed, Paracelsianism then spread elsewhere in translations in Latin and other languages, as well as through the works of his followers. Despite resistance by various medical establishments that remained wedded to humoralism, Paracelsian chemical medicine became increasingly popular across Western Europe, from which it spread to the European colonies overseas such as the Spanish colony of Mexico, as well as other regions, notably the Ottoman Empire.[5] Some of the physicians imported by the Apothecary Chancery brought Paracelsian ideas with them, linking the Russian Empire to both the long-term global practice of medical chemistry and the contemporary international argument over the value of Paracelsianism.

In contrast to the well-documented history of chemical medicine elsewhere, the evidence for Russian chemical medicine is ambivalent. Historians arguing that chemical medicine was used by the Russian court in the sixteenth century have primarily relied upon modern autopsies of court figures that reveal excess levels of mercury and other chemicals in those bodies, yet that evidence can be interpreted variously.[6] The Slavonic version of the princely manual *Secretum secretorum* does include sections on chemicals, but those have been garbled in translation.[7] Most importantly, none of the extant sixteenth-century prescriptions list known terms for chemicals.[8] The surviving traces of official Russian medicine from the sixteenth century do not attest to a chemical medical tradition.

This absence of chemical ingredients in the traces of official Russian medicine in the sixteenth century both continued and evolved in the early seventeenth century. Extant prescriptions from the first half of the century lack Paracelsian ingredients like mercury and arsenic. More importantly, a version of the Apothecary Chancery oath from the 1640s includes an imprecation not to prescribe "chemical preparations" [*khimicheskie preparati*], indicating not merely a disinterest in chemical medicine, but an active hostility towards it on the part of the Russian administrators who created and administered that oath.[9] Yet there were chemically inclined practitioners associated with the court in the early seventeenth century, at least one of whom tried to get Russian officials on side for chemical medicine with a written defence of the practice. The picture that emerges of the status of chemical medicine at the Russian court before the mid-seventeenth century is of some support for chemical medicine among medical practitioners that was stymied by disinterest or hostility towards those materials by court officials.

In the second half of the century, things began to change. There was a gradual shift in prescription practices, with more chemicals emerging. Chemicals also began to appear in official books, like the *pharmacopoeia* of the Apothecary Chancery. This was linked to the activities of the medical practitioners: in this period, they switched back to writing chemical medical tracts aimed at patrons that specifically argued for the inclusion of chemical medicine in the category of good drugs. All was not plain sailing. In the 1690s, there was an argument over the value of Padua graduates specifically referencing a supposed lack of a chemical education in that university. Medical practitioners considered this a problem; Russian officials disregarded the advice and hired the Padua graduates anyway. Despite this ongoing reluctance of Russian officials to seriously consider the merits of chemical medicine, official records of inventories and prescriptions show an uptick in the kinds of chemicals being used in the late seventeenth and early eighteenth centuries.

This debate over chemicals as *materia medica* between Western European physicians and Russian officials shows a form of regulatory co-construction. Kapil Raj has used the term "co-construction" to refer to the creation of knowledge texts, arguing that different groups in both South Asia and Europe contributed to the construction of knowledge texts by providing different kinds of expertise.[10] Such co-construction of texts was common, especially in colonial contexts, such as the 1613 *Confessionario,* conventionally solely attributed to the Spaniard Francisco Pareja, but linguistic analysis of which has shown it to have been co-produced by Pareja and at least two speakers of the Native American language Timucua.[11] This form of hidden co-construction also shows up elsewhere in early modern science, such as with the British chemist Robert Boyle's reliance upon technicians who get little credit in his published work.[12] In the various sites of early modern science and medicine, it was entirely standard for knowledge to be constructed between multiple groups, as they all learned from each other, and had to take account of each other, even when the final text either does not explicitly acknowledge, or in fact actively seeks to conceal, that co-construction.

The Russian case shows that not just knowledge but also rules were co-constructed. In the Apothecary Chancery both the chemically inclined and the chemical skeptics worked for the same institution and had to take account of one another. At the start of the seventeenth century, there was a gulf between foreign medical practitioners and Russian officials: the former wanted to use chemicals in medicines; the latter did not. Across the century, the medical practitioners made their case and gained ground, creating a new co-constructed set of norms regarding drug making. The international connections of the Moscow court meant that in the Apothecary Chancery medical practitioners from Western Europe and Russian officials came together to negotiate over the rules of drug construction. Neither group could operate without the co-operation of the other, and so rules had to be co-constructed between the different groups in order to work.

PARACELSIAN *APOLOGIA*

From the very start of the seventeenth century, texts were being produced in Russia promoting the virtues of chemical medicine. Those texts either were written by figures linked to official Russian medicine or were addressed to significant figures in the Russian elite. They were written by Western Europeans, one group within the hybrid institution of the Apothecary Chancery and the diverse ecosystem of medical knowledge and expertise on the natural world within the Russian Empire. Like their contemporaries in both Western Europe and the Ottoman Empire, from the very start of the seventeenth century certain medical practitioners in Moscow were promoting the new, Paracelsian, chemical medicine.

One important text here is a letter written in 1626 by the Dutchman Gerard von der Geiden to Tsar Mikhail Fedorovich; the missive concerns alchemy. This document, which runs to several pages, covers not only the Philosophers' Stone – the major goal of the alchemists, a substance said to allow the transmutation of lead into gold and grant eternal life – but also how to use metals and chemicals for a variety of purposes, including medicine. Significantly, von der Geiden recommends the use of mercury for internal medicine.[13] Mercury, also known under its early modern name of quicksilver, is a highly toxic heavy metal the use of which in internal medicines was central to Paracelsian medicine for a range of ailments, and was also commonly used by various early modern medical practitioners as a treatment for syphilis. Von der Geiden certainly believed that the early seventeenth-century Russian court should practise chemical medicine, including the fundamentals of Paracelsian practice.

Von der Geiden's text, which includes comments on the philosophers' stone, chemical medicine, and other uses of chemicals, comes across as a rather eclectic document. Such a broad view of the uses of chemicals fits well with recent histories of alchemy. Previously, much attention had been devoted to the philosophical side of that art, which was important to alchemy, but not the entirety of what early modern European alchemy was. As shown by scholars like William Newman and Lawrence Principe, there was always a distinctly practical side to alchemy in early modern Europe, whether about medicine, mining, or metalwork, a side in part deliberately obscured by practitioners themselves, as they hid trade secrets behind grand metaphor, and in part later consciously misinterpreted by early modern chemists like the British Robert Boyle, who took the best of the alchemists' work as their own while denigrating their legacy.[14] Von der Geiden's letter to the tsar bridges those traditions, being both practical and philosophical.

Particularly significant for our purposes here is von der Geiden's interest in chemicals in medicine, medicine for the elite, and internal medicine. The Russian response to von der Geiden's letter – if there was one – has not survived. Yet fundamentally the letter itself represents a consideration of the limitations of appropriate medicines, in this case where chemical medicines should fit within that project. Von der Geiden was arguing for the use of Paracelsian medicine for the court, including the use of such notable substances as mercury. The Russian elite of the early seventeenth century were then aware of chemical medicine and had opportunities to consider bringing it into practice as a part of official medicine, but there is no direct evidence that von der Geiden's chemical proposal was taken up.

Another figure associated with the early seventeenth-century Russian court who had certainly the knowledge and perhaps the will to engage in chemical medicine was Arthur Dee (in Russia 1621–34). Arthur Dee was the son of the famous Elizabethan magus John Dee, inventor (or discoverer) of the Enochian Angel language, and court astrologer and alchemist to the Holy Roman Emperor Rudolph II.[15] Dee shared his father's occult leanings. As an adult, Dee took up some of father's passions, writing a treatise called *Chemical Collections* [*Fasciculus chemicus*] in the early 1630s when he was in Moscow, using books he had with him there in his private library.[16] As the title suggests, this work was specifically focused on the uses of chemicals. Dee's work gathers together quotations and thoughts from various chemical thinkers, including thoughts on chemical medicine.[17] Like von der Geiden, Dee specifically recommends the use of mercury in medical drugs.[18] Dee was certainly engaged with chemical medicine during his stay in Muscovy, advocating to his readers the value of mercury as *materia medica.*

The relationship between Dee's work at court and the creation of the *Chemical Collections* is unclear. His work is linked to the Russian court as the book proclaims itself to be "the work and study of Arthur Dee, chief physician of the Tsar of all the Russias," a phrase later paralleled by another Apothecary Chancery employee, Daniel Gurchin, who referred to himself in a similar fashion in his early eighteenth-century works specifically aimed at a Russian-speaking Moscow-based audience.[19] Yet this phrase alone is insufficient to determine that Dee was seeking a Russian readership. Dee wrote in Latin, and there are later editions of his work in English, but no Russian version has ever been identified. It was only in the eighteenth century that works began to be produced in Latin for a Russian audience.[20] There were few Muscovites who read Latin in the first half of the seventeenth century, so Dee was likely seeking a Western European rather than a Russian audience. Dee had closer links to official Russian medicine than van der Geiden, but he did not use those links to present his book on chemicals to a Russian audience.

From the start of the seventeenth century, certain figures based in Moscow and with links to the Russian elite were convinced of the value of chemical medicine. They expressed their interest in it via written works, one directly addressed to the Russian court, one not. Both works specifically promote the use of mercury, considered so important by Paracelsians, as an ingredient for medical drugs. The Russian court were then certainly in a position to be aware of the new interest in chemical medicine, as they were aware of the new enthusiasm for American medicinal plants around the same period. Yet unlike the eager uptake of American medicinal plants, the acceptance of chemicals as medicine in Russia would be slower and more complicated.

CHEMICAL ABSENCES

Van der Geiden and Dee, residents of Moscow with strong links to the court, approved of chemical medicine. Yet this approval did not initially translate into practice. Van der Geiden never worked for the Apothecary Chancery, and there is evidence that suggests that Dee did not practise chemical medicine within the department. Here, we have both positive and negative evidence. The positive evidence is an oath from the 1640s specifically restricting the use of chemical medicines; the negative evidence is the very limited quantity and variety of chemicals found in extant documents from the first half of the seventeenth century. The second type of evidence is troublesome. Absence of evidence, as we know, is not evidence of absence. Yet it is still significant. If chemical medicine were a major or even regular part of practice in the Apothecary Chancery in the early seventeenth century we should be able to find some evidence for it, and likely of the *tria prima* that were so key to Paracelsus's practice: salt, sulphur, and mercury. Yet these ingredients are hard to find in Apothecary Chancery documents. Despite the presence of chemical practitioners at the court in the early seventeenth century, what we find in the Apothecary Chancery is closer to an absence of chemical medicine.

The most explicit piece of evidence regarding the Apothecary Chancery's stance on chemical medicine comes, as usual, from the oaths. Around a decade after Dee composed his chemical work, the Apothecary Chancery oath banned the use of "chemical preparations" [*khimicheskie preparati*] as internal consumable medicines.[21] The text itself gives no specifics as to what counts as a chemical preparation, nor any justification for that prohibition. Given the prominence of Paracelsian chemical medicine in the Western European medical circles from which the court recruited their physicians, we can hypothesize that the department was banning some, or perhaps even all, of the substances of Paracelsian chemical medicine, including the *tria prima*. Something chemical was limited for some period around the 1640s. But the specific limits and reasons for that are not clear from the oath alone.

Yet these two words are still significant. Inclusion of a prohibition in an oath is serious business. Oaths had the force of law. Breaking any part of the oath was strictly punished, as the internal Apothecary Chancery investigations we looked at in chapter 1 demonstrate. So, the restriction on chemical preparations should be considered a notable part of early seventeenth-century official Russian medicine. Conversely, we have only one extant manuscript that includes the phrase banning chemical preparations. Manuscript survival is always tricky. The number of surviving copies of certain kinds of texts is always lower than the number of copies that actually existed, yet by how much is always unclear. A limited number of extant copies can mean a limited number were created, or it can mean a large number were created and were in such heavy use that many fell apart from use. In the case of the oaths, we have some indications of a high attrition rate. Every Apothecary Chancery servitor was required to take the oath, meaning hundreds of oath-taking ceremonies across the century. Yet only a handful of manuscripts survive. We have, necessarily, lost a lot. The ban on using chemical preparations in Apothecary Chancery medicines was broader than the manuscript survival can directly attest.

Here we can turn to the other documents of the Apothecary Chancery, like import lists, inventories, and prescriptions, to contextualize the 1640s oath. If chemicals were generally used in the early seventeenth century and the oath is an aberration, we should find some evidence of chemicals, perhaps even substantial evidence of them. Conversely, if we find no or limited evidence of chemicals in this period, we can take the oath as more typical of the overall official medical culture of the period. As a point of comparison, the first *Pharmacopoeia* (list of approved medicines) to include chemical medicine as a major category was the 1618 *Pharmacopoeia Londinensis,* which listed eighty-five chemical preparations including twenty kinds of "chemical oil" as well as multiple compounds of mercury and antimony.[22] We can compare the extant traces of chemical medicine in official Russian medicine to this quantity of approved chemical medicines from contemporary England to see where Russia measured up in its use of chemical medicines.

One significant group of documents are the import lists, records of what the Apothecary Chancery purchased from Western European markets. These are often long and detailed documents recording hundreds of ingredients for medicines alongside other supplies such as various kinds of equipment. As we saw in chapter 2, plants were a regular and substantial part of those import lists. Finding chemicals in these documents is much harder. The earliest extant import list, from 1602, does include chemical substances: two kinds of sulphur – sulphur citrinum and *flores sulphuris* – as well as the mineral borax, and vitriol.[23] The latter could be one of several materials, a sulphate of iron, copper, magnesium or zinc; it was commonly used in Paracelsian medicine, and was also an ingredient in the philosopher's stone.[24] Of the 164 items on that list, four are chemicals, but only one of the *tria prima* is listed. Both of the other imports from before 1650, a 1645 import from Hamburg, and a 1647 import from Amsterdam, include vitriol as their only chemical item, and none of the *tria prima*.[25] During the first half of the seventeenth century, the Apothecary Chancery purchase records show a very limited range of chemicals being imported, and the *tria prima* in particular have a minimal presence.

Prescription documents tell a similar story. In the ten extant prescriptions from 1629–33 only vitriol is listed, and only once.[26] The next set of prescriptions that survive are twenty-four such documents from 1643–45; those do not list the *tria prima* but they do include two uses of vitriol.[27] Vitriol was prescribed at least twice more in the first half of the seventeenth century.[28] Another chemical occasionally prescribed in this period was antimony, a metalloid recommended by Paracelsus as a laxative and by other chemical authors as a purgative.[29] Prescriptions then generally echo the import records in their limited record of chemicals in general and the near-total absence of the *tria prima* in particular.

As well as prescribing to the courtly elite, the Apothecary Chancery also sent out medicines to the army. Before 1650, we have four such lists specifying what was provided: all of them are from 1633. All four include vitriol on their list, and one *plaster stiptikum*.[30] This is a reference to the so-called Paracelsus Plaster, also known as *Emplastrum stipticum Paracelsi*, a medicine associated by name (if in reality probably not created by) the great chemical medical thinker himself.[31] The recipe was well known in Western Europe from at least the early seventeenth century.[32] An early eighteenth-century version of this recipe lists its ingredients as oil of olives, yellow wax, litharge [lead monoxide], gum ammoniacum, bdellium [a kind of gum resin from South Asia], galbanum [a kind of gum resin from Persia], opoponax [a kind of gum resin from East Africa], oil of bays, calamine, birthwort, myrrh, frankincense, and turpentine.[33] So, a medicine linked by name to the major proponent of chemical medicine did not contain chemicals. Among the medical supplies of the Russian army before 1650 we find some small traces of chemical medicine in the form of one chemical and one mostly herbal medicament linked to chemical medicine by the name of a practitioner alone.

We can compare these limited chemical provisions for the army to prescriptions for the more elite patients of the court. Here, we have thirty-six prescriptions across the 1630s and 1640s, of which five include a chemical of some kind; three specify vitriol, two the Paracelsus plaster, and one other antimony.[34] We have only a fragmented survival of prescriptions and army lists from the first decades of the seventeenth century, so this is certainly not a complete picture of the official prescribing practices of the period, but it is suggestive. There could have been other chemicals in use in this period, but the absence of them in extant documents suggests that this would have at most been an occasional practice. Before 1650, there was limited use of chemicals in the Apothecary Chancery for all kinds of patients, and no extant prescription mentions any of the *tria prima*.

We then need to understand what motivated the Apothecary Chancery to limit and at times reject this category of drugs. We should remember here that opinions in Western Europe were divided on the utility of chemical medicine, and it is likely that some of the Apothecary Chancery's physicians were keener on these substances than others. Medical practitioners across Western Europe clashed over the validity of chemical medicine, including in England and the Germans Lands, two of the department's key recruiting grounds.[35] Some Apothecary Chancery physicians would likely have followed van der Geiden and Dee in their enthusiasm for chemical medicine; others would probably have been more circumspect.

Even more significant was the view of the Russian administrators of the department. The Apothecary Chancery was always under the control of a Russian noble, who was helped and advised by Russian administrators. As we saw in chapter 1, the Russian court was extremely concerned about poisonings, a concern only heightened by the rumoured poisonings of multiple key figures during the Time of Troubles at the start of the seventeenth century. An alternate theory for the mercury that modern autopsies found in the remains of certain Russian royals and nobles who died in this period is that this is evidence of poisoning, not of chemical medicine.[36] Whether or not those people were in fact killed with these specific substances, both arsenic and mercury were well known as poisons across early modern Europe.[37] All of this points to certain materials of chemical medicine, notably arsenic and mercury, having the reputation of poisons in seventeenth-century Russia, a fact that could have motivated restricting their use in medicines.

The restriction on using chemical preparations as medicines found in the 1640s Apothecary Chancery oath was then not absolute. The department imported, stocked, and prescribed some chemicals in the first half of the seventeenth century, sending those medicines both to low-status patients like the army and high-status patients like members of court. Yet the quantities and varieties of chemicals are distinctly limited: vitriol was the near-exclusive focus of this practice; Paracelsus's *tria prima* were all but totally absent. There was some use of chemical medicine, but substantially fewer kinds of chemical medicines were purchased or created than the eighty-five found in the 1618 *Pharmacopoeia Londinensis*. Perhaps motivated by fears of poisoning, official Russian medicine of the early seventeenth century allowed much less space for chemical medicines than official British medicine. Despite the enthusiasm for Paracelsianism on the part of certain medical practitioners in early seventeenth-century Moscow, the Apothecary Chancery was not a chemical medical institution in the first half of the seventeenth century.

CHEMICAL MEDICINE RISING

When the Apothecary Chancery restricted chemical medicines in the early seventeenth century, they were going against a trend that had spread across Western Europe, Western Europe's overseas colonies, and the Ottoman Empire, as well as against the views of some of the department's own medical practitioners. This was not unusual behaviour for the department. We saw in chapter 1 how medical practice in the Apothecary Chancery was regulated by oaths based on Muscovite practices, not Western European norms. Foreign medical practitioners were important to the work of the department, but they worked for the Russian bureaucrats. However, the bureaucrats who controlled official Russian medicine could only exercise so much influence over their medical practitioners. Looking past the 1640s oath into the second half of the seventeenth century we see that there was a gradual uptick in the use of chemical medicines, a trend that we can link to the activities of Apothecary Chancery medical practitioners.

In the first half of the seventeenth century, we found only a handful of chemicals in medical use; in the second half of the century that number began slowly to rise. We see the same ingredients as we saw in the first half of the seventeenth century in the second half of that century. An inventory compiled sometime in the 1660s–1680s includes antimony, vitriol, and borax.[38] A collection of thirty prescriptions from 1667–74 includes one reference to vitriol.[39] Similarly, a collection of thirty prescriptions from 1673–74 lists only vitriol, once.[40] A collection of five prescriptions from 1682 lists saltpetre once.[41] From the 1660s to the 1680s, we see the limited quantity of materials we saw earlier being kept in stock and in use in this later period.

We also see other chemical ingredients start to appear in the records in this period. In the prescriptions from 1667 to 1674, we also find one instance of sal ammoniac, a mineral.[42] The five prescriptions from 1682 also list sal ammoniac once.[43] Ninety-three prescriptions from 1698 include sulphur and ammoniac, as well as four instances of the symbol for mercury.[44] Arsenic, sometimes used for chemical medicine in Western Europe, appears only in late seventeenth-century Apothecary Chancery records as a poison.[45] By the end of the seventeenth century, we see a greater range of chemicals being kept in stock and being prescribed by the department, including the use of Paracelsus's *tria prima.*

The use of these chemicals was still limited compared with the botanicals, the Apothecary Chancery's favourite category of ingredient. In the collection of prescriptions from 1667 to 1674, there is one mention of vitriol, and one of ammoniac, whereas senna is listed three times and nutmeg four.[46] The collection of five prescriptions from 1682 lists sal ammoniac and saltpetre once each, as opposed to four mentions of nutmeg.[47] The 1698 prescription collection has four uses of the symbol for mercury; the same set of recipes lists sassafras and sarsaparilla three times each.[48] That still-limited range of chemicals is prescribed generally less frequently than other ingredients, including plants grown far from the Russian Empire, like nutmeg or sassafras. There are more chemicals being prescribed in the late seventeenth century than in the early part of the century, but the quantity of chemical ingredients being used does not come close to the huge volume of plants, and also remained substantially limited compared with the use of chemicals elsewhere.

We find a more dramatic change in the status of chemical medicines when we look at official Russian medical texts from this period. One work in particular is vital here: the Apothecary Chancery *Pharmacopoeia.* This work, the compiler of which T.V. Panich has identified as Daniel Gurchin, then an apothecary in the Apothecary Chancery, was initially translated from an as-yet-unidentified Latin pharmacy work in 1676.[49] It was then copied and adapted over the next several decades, with the main extant manuscript dating to 1700. This text may be what Peter Burke, following

Michel Garneau, refers to as a "tradaption," a work listed as a translation but which was substantially adapted in translation.[50] As well as the translation of the Latin text, the 1700 manuscript collects together Apothecary Chancery recipes and notes on treatment from as early as the 1650s, and as late as the 1700s. We can then see this text as a history of late seventeenth-century Russian medicine in and of itself, a history in which, crucially, we find chemical medicine.

The main section of the manuscript, the section around which all the other parts were constructed, is a *Pharmacopoeia* text, identified only from the following statement: "Pharmacopoeia on the preparations of medicines, translated from Latin into Slavonic AD 1676."[51] The text gives no other clue as to its origin. The text following this heading consists of recipes organized by type of medicine, with recipes for plasters, ointments, powders, syrups, sugars, oils, vodkas, elixirs, and other alcoholic spirits.[52] The text recommends the use of multiple chemical ingredients in these recipes, including mercury, sulphur, sal ammoniac, and saltpetre, plus the Paracelsus Plaster.[53] The main text of the Apothecary Chancery *Pharmacopoeia* was then a text that recommended chemicals in medicine, including the Paracelsian *tria prima*.

Looking at the additional recipes included in the 1700 copy of the *Pharmacopoeia*, we can see more chemical medicine. Interestingly, these recipes are linked to specific named Apothecary Chancery practitioners, indicating that the practitioner prescribed that specific recipe. An undated recipe by Johann Guttmensch, who worked in the Apothecary Chancery between 1668 and 1682,[54] goes as follows:

> *Spiritus Salis Ammoniacum* is composed as follows.
> Mix together sal ammoniac, lime, and red vitriol with fresh, clean woman's water [*sic*] and leave to stand for 2 to 3 days in a closed vessel, and after that stir all of it into a different vessel filtering it [lit. cleanly] through grey paper and be careful to close the vessel firmly. And you can inhale this [mixture] for head pain and closed nostrils.[55]

Guttmensch here then specifically prescribed medicines partly composed of chemicals. Other Apothecary Chancery medical practitioners also contributed additional recipes containing chemicals to the manuscript: Stefan von Gaden, who worked in the department from 1657 until his death in 1682, provided two that recommended the use of sal ammoniac.[56] The chemical aspects of the Apothecary Chancery *Pharmacopoeia* can thus be partly linked to certain practitioners within the department who practised a form of chemical medicine.

The 1676 Apothecary Chancery *Pharmacopoeia* was one of a number of works owned or created by the department. According to the carefully reconstructed yet incomplete book list compiled by E.A. Savel'eva, by the late seventeenth century the department had a fairly extensive library, including many texts on medicine and natural philosophy.[57] Indeed, this period saw serious text acquisition, translation, and copying in the Apothecary Chancery. Only four years previous to the Apothecary Chancery *Pharmacopoeia*'s compilation in 1676, that other major medical text for early modern Russia, the *Garden of Health*, was recopied.[58] Apothecary Chancery documents testify to several other individual medical works being translated.[59] Among the works owned by the Apothecary Chancery were chemical medical texts such as Johann Schröder's 1644 *Pharmocopoeia medicochymica* and Johannes Daniel Hortius's 1651 *Pharmacopoiea Galeno-Chemica.*[60] In the same period in which the Apothecary Chancery was prescribing a greater quantity and variety of chemical medicines, it was also acquiring a number of chemical medical works.

Comparing the extant documentary traces of chemical medicine in official Russian medical sources from the early to the late seventeenth century we see a change. In the early part of the century, we find few mentions of chemicals, almost entirely restricted to vitriol. We also find the oath that specifically restricts the use of chemicals. Documents from the second half of the century show the use of a greater variety of chemicals, including the use of Paracelsus's *tria prima*. The 1700 copy of the Apothecary Chancery *Pharmacopoeia* also contains a variety of chemicals; that work was one of several owned by the Apothecary Chancery in the late seventeenth century that related to chemical medicine. Also significantly, the Apothecary Chancery *Pharmacopoeia* contains recipes linking chemical medicine to specific practitioners within the department. By the end of the century, the Apothecary Chancery's use of chemicals was more substantial than it had been at the start of the century, and there is reason to link that shift to the medical practitioners of the department.

THE PADUA QUESTION

A different measure of the rising importance of chemical medicine in late seventeenth-century official Russian medicine, and one that underlines the significance of the department's medical practitioners in this process, comes from a report written in 1690. For some decades, it had been the department's practice to examine certain new recruits on their medical knowledge. The earliest exam was of the British physician Timothy Willis in 1599; the department continued to periodically require such exams for potential recruits who for one reason or another raised some suspicion over their suitability until at least 1702, when Doctor Gliusnik presented a copy of his doctoral thesis on dysentery during his hiring process.[61] In 1690, the department decided that it needed a background report on the alma mater of some potential recruits, a certain university of Padua. The resulting report specifically highlighted the question of chemical medicine in the training of physicians.

The author of the report – Laurentius Blumentrost senior, a German, and then one of the Apothecary Chancery's top physicians – declared that Padua thoroughly prepares its students in the ancient works of Galen, whose writings are essential to medical practice: students of Padua can recite Galen's works accurately and are also learned in the proper application of venesection to regulate humours [here *vlazhebniki,* pl.; *vlazhebnik,* sing.], a practice that can be dangerous if improperly used. Stressing the central role knowledge of Galen and humours play in contemporary medicine, Blumentrost notes that knowledge of such matters is essential to becoming a physician.[62] Padua was thus judged to be a good university by Blumentrost inasfar as it trained its students in the use of Galenic medicine.

The Galenic medicine and humours to which Blumentrost here refers would have been familiar to the Muscovite readers of his report. Not only did a humoral understanding of the body come up in earlier Apothecary Chancery reports, such as that on the final illness of Mikhail Fedorovich (see chapter 2), but other texts circulating the pre-modern East Slavic lands also mentioned humours. Sviatoslav's Miscellany [*Izbornik Sviatoslava*] of 1073 stated that "it is said the human body therefore is composed of four parts. It has warmth from [the element of] fire, cold from wind, dryness from earth, moisture from water."[63] We see a similar sentiment in Pseudi-Galen's "Galen on Hippocrates," which circulated in pre-modern Russia in medical miscellanies well into the eighteenth century. Pseudo-Galen tells us that "The world is composed of four things. From fire. From air. From earth. From water."[64] Blumentrost, in praising Galenic humoralism, was dealing with a subject familiar to educated Russians.

In contrast to his praise for Padua's Galenic credentials, Blumentrost criticized Padua for its approach to other medical practices. According to Blumentrost, Padua defames Paracelsus and Jan Baptist von Helmont, the controversial leading figures of chemical medicine. Worse still, to Blumentrost's thinking, is Padua's rejection of the chemical elements present in ancient authors, in particular the respected Hippocrates but also Plato, whom Blumentrost also includes in the ranks of the chemically minded. Blumentrost states that

> in Italy those [ideas concerning chemical medicine] are not put to [the test of] fire and water, [as the Italians] fear deeply concealed nature, and [so reject] the most tolerable teaching concerning fermentation not only of Paracelsus or [von] Helmont but also [that of] the great Hippocrates, Plato and other most ancient teachers, whom are now and from ancient [times] accepted and respected.[65]

Blumentrost thus endorsed Padua as a centre of medical learning, and so the value of degrees issued by that institution, but also warned that the knowledge gained there was incomplete as the Italians would not give a fair hearing to chemical medicine.

This concern about the reception of chemical medicine in Padua by a German seems to have been rooted in a genuine disconnection between northern Europe and Italy over the value of the chemical tradition. A seventeenth-century Pisan official noted that it was hard to introduce chemistry and chemical medicine into Italian universities, as the Paracelsians were "damned in all [Italian] universities," in part because of a preference for the Mechanists, those early modern European thinkers who believed the universe could be understood as a collection of mechanical principles.[66] In contrast, Antonio Clericuzio has stated that Helmontian chemical medicine did enjoy some success in Italy, but primarily in Venice and Naples.[67] There may have been some truth in Blumentrost's complaints that Padua did not take chemical medicine seriously.

Paracelsus and von Helmont, the chemical medical practitioners Blumentrost defended, were, respectively, from Switzerland and the Netherlands, and so were also northern Europeans. Paracelsus in particular was both a controversial and an almost revered figure. His works were originally composed in German, and Latin translations, the usual language of scholarship in Western Europe, were late and rare. In this respect Paracelsus has been compared to Martin Luther, who had been the first man to write theology in German; Paracelsus was the first to write a scientific text in German. Paracelsus's work was then bound up with a burgeoning German vernacular identity.[68] The absence of these men's work from the curriculum of an Italian university was an insult to German medical science. In defending Paracelsus, and his other fellow northern European von Helmont, Blumentrost was defending his linguistic identity. Moreover, he was explicitly locating chemical medicine firmly within the boundaries of acceptable medical practice of the 1690s.

Blumentrost was convinced of the value of chemical medicine and of the problems with Paduan medical education. His attempt to convince his employers of this was not successful, as the doctors Blumentrost examined were hired despite his reservations. Also interestingly, the report on Padua was composed just two years before the first Russian to successfully study abroad, Petr Postnikov, was sent to none other than the medical faculty of the university of Padua. Postnikov's biographer Dmitrii Tsvetaev makes much of the decision to send Postnikov to an Italian university rather than one of the German universities that supplied so many of the Apothecary Chancery's physicians in the late seventeenth century. Indeed, Tsvetaev claims, German physicians' resentment over Postnikov's alma mater was one reason Postnikov spent little time working in the Apothecary Chancery, being quickly transferred to the Ambassadorial Chancery and working as a diplomat for most of his years of service.[69] Following Postnikov, Peter the Great later sent a further sixty Russians abroad to study in 1697, forty of whom were sent to Italy (the rest went to the Netherlands).[70] Blumentrost's complaints about the Italians' opposition to chemical medicine did not affect the decisions of the Russian administrators regarding hiring and training medical practitioners.

By the 1690s, chemical medicine was more accepted within the Apothecary Chancery than it had been in the 1640s. More chemicals were being prescribed, chemical medical books were purchased and composed, and chemical medicine was defended in a report. Significantly, this pro-chemical medicine activity can be linked to the medical practitioners of the department like Guttmensch, von Gaden, and Blumentrost. In contrast, Russian bureaucrats were at best indifferent to chemical medicine. As late as the 1690s, chemical medicine was not fully endorsed by the Russian elite, and it was foreign medical practitioners who were pushing for it to be accepted.

FOLLOWING THE DOCTORS

From the 1690s on, certain medical practitioners in Russia tried to promote chemical medicine through texts, partly through reports for the Apothecary Chancery, but also increasingly through books aimed at specific patrons. This strategy involved a broader collection of medical experts than before. Two major figures in this part of the story are Apothecary Chancery employees, and men whose enthusiasm for chemical medicine we have already seen: the apothecary Daniel Gurchin and the physician Laurentius Blumentrost; a third was the churchman Archbishop Afanasii of Kholmogory. Between them, they created several chemical medical texts in the late seventeenth century that continued to be copied into the eighteenth century. Following their work in the 1690s, eighteenth-century Russian medicine, both official and unofficial, used chemical medicine much more extensively than it had in the previous century. After internal debate within the Apothecary Chancery, returning to the tactics used by van der Geiden in the 1620s and more directly addressing elite patrons took the Russian chemical medical movement to something like success.

This success was made at the intersection of several spheres of Muscovite medicine. The most immediate one was the intersection between court medicine and religious healing. This intersection produced the *Extract from Doctors' Knowledge* [*Reestr iz dokhturskikh nauk*], a medical recipe book first created in the 1690s but copied many times in the late seventeenth and into the eighteenth century. The text was a collaboration between an Apothecary Chancery employee and a churchman. This immediately crosses a notable line in Muscovite medicine, from secular to religious medicine. Although there were some formal links between the Apothecary Chancery and the church – the department provided supplies for the church to make holy *miro* – their medical practices were separate.[71] Kholmogory was part of a group of churchmen who saw medicaments as a part of God's plan and had peppered the natural world with useful remedies for humanity's ailments. It was this view of religious healing that led Kholmogory to link up his faith-based healing with the object-based secular healing of the Apothecary Chancery.

The *Extract from Doctors' Knowledge*, compiled in 1696 by Archbishop Afanasii of Kholmogory and Apothecary Chancery apothecary Daniel Gurchin, was created on the basis of the Apothecary Chancery *Pharmacopoeia*, itself a creation of Gurchin.[72] Indeed, there is such a high degree of similarity between the texts that T.V. Panich considers the *Extract from Doctors' Knowledge* a variant text of the *Pharmacopoeia*.[73] As such, the *Extract from Doctors' Knowledge* contains much of the same pharmaceutical knowledge about complex recipes and the preparation of medicines that was included in the *Pharmacopoeia*. Like the Apothecary Chancery *Pharmacopoeia*, the *Extract from Doctors' Knowledge* also included chemicals, notably two of the *tria prima* sulphur and mercury.[74] This collaboration between secular and religious medicine was in part a chemical collaboration.

We can further examine the *Extract from Doctors' Knowledge* chemical leanings by looking at a recipe in detail. The thirtieth (of fifty-five) recipes goes as follows:

> Recipe for an ointment for itches is to be made in the following way. Take fresh inula, onion, as much as you like, chop up, and put in cow's butter, so that the ratio of butter to onion is 1:2, and add a handful of inula [and] salt, a handful of sulphur. And cook together, until steam appears, then take it off the fire, strain through a cloth onto a wooden plate or into a vessel. And to that mixture add mercury, and mix, until the mercury dies [*sic*], and the ointment turns dark blue.
>
> And rub that ointment onto itchy places – it will dry and revive [them].[75]

This recipe demonstrates two significant points. The *Extract from Doctors' Knowledge* uses mercury, a substance not in use by the Apothecary Chancery until the second half of the seventeenth century. And we can see in one recipe the use of two different chemicals, mercury and sulphur. The *Extract from Doctors' Knowledge* then followed the late seventeenth century trend towards increasing use of chemicals in medicines.

In its content, the *Extract from Doctors' Knowledge* took much from the Apothecary Chancery *Pharmacopoeia*; in its audience it was very different. The *Pharmacopoeia* was created for and used by trained medical practitioners in the Apothecary Chancery. The original *Extract from Doctors' Knowledge* was aimed at a single lay patron, Fedor Matveevich Apraksin, military governor [*voevoda*] of Dvina, a district near that of Afanasii's archbishopric of Kholmogory. Both were located in northern Russia, along the trade route to the major seventeenth-century entrepôt of Archangel, the landing place for so many of the foreign substances – and foreign medical practitioners – who entered Muscovy. Apraksin was linked to the Moscow court; his position as governor was a state responsibility, and he was in constant correspondence with the Kremlin. Nevertheless, his office and home were hundreds of miles to the northeast of the Apothecary Chancery. The *Extract from Doctors' Knowledge* promoted chemical medicine not only outside of official medical circles, but to a patron physically very distant from the home of official Muscovite medicine in Moscow.

The *Extract from Doctors' Knowledge* sat on the boundary of secular and religious medicine; two years later, the prolific Gurchin collaborated on another text, one that sat on the boundary of official and lay medicine. In the 1690s, Gurchin and Laurentius Blumentrost senior created the royal version of the *Domestic and Field Pharmacy,* in part on the basis of Blumentrost's 1667 *Pharmacotheca domestica et portatilis.* The original was given to Tsar Peter the Great, and the text was later reproduced for his son, Tsarevich Aleksei.[76] This text, the main part of which is a medical recipe book, contains chemical ingredients, including sulphur and sal ammoniac. One chapter is on mercury.[77] Like the *Extract from Doctors' Knowledge,* the royal *Domestic and Field Pharmacy* explicitly recommended the use of chemicals in medicine.

The royal *Domestic and Field Pharmacy* is also significant to the history of chemical medicine in Russia as it gives us the most direct and uncompromising statement of support for chemical medicine. The introduction to this text states "I have always honoured chemical and apothecary science since my youth."[78] This is a startling statement for a Muscovite document. As we have seen, Russian texts of this period often express themselves obliquely, and the medical texts in particular commonly present recipes rather than clear statements of affiliation to a particular medical philosophy. We see here confirmation of Gurchin's and Blumentrost's interests in chemical medicine that we had already discerned from their other writings. And we see that they directed their most explicit statement of his chemical medical affiliation towards a major patron with the power to reshape official medical practice. In addressing the tsar personally with their extended chemical *apologia*, Gurchin and Blumentrost were doing more than recommending a set of treatments for an individual; they were proposing a program for the medical development of the whole country.

Gurchin would continue his creation of texts containing chemical medical recipes in the eighteenth century.[79] He would revise the *Domestic and Field Pharmacy* presented to Peter into a text for a non-elite audience.[80] He also compiled the *Pharmacy for Transport or Service*, a text aimed at soldiers and other servitors that includes recipes with chemical ingredients such as saltpetre. One manuscript of that text contains a recipe headed "chemical medicine" [*meditsyna khimika*], explicitly stating a chemical medical approach.[81] Another of Gurchin's creations was the *Small Domestic Pharmacy*, which similarly includes multiple chemicals.[82] Gurchin's works were not the only Russian-language medical works that were aimed at a lay readership and promoted the use of chemicals in medicine in the eighteenth century. The 1730 *Little Ark of Medicine* [*Kovchezhets meditsinskii*] includes a similar mix of chemical and compound medicine, such as the "Paracelsus elixir."[83] By the mid-eighteenth century, a number of works were circulating the Russian Empire that promoted chemical medicine to a lay readership.

As chemical and pharmaceutical medicine was being promoted in books aimed at lay audiences, it was also increasingly being practised in official medicine. The inventories of the Medical Chancellery are revealing. Vitriol, previously used by the Apothecary Chancery, was regularly in stock.[84] Mercury, which the Apothecary Chancery did not use before the 1690s, appears in six inventories in the 1730s and 1750s.[85] Even arsenic, only referred to in Apothecary Chancery records as a poison, appears in one such inventory from 1738 of supplies for the Moscow main pharmacy and a local hospital.[86] Lists of materials sent to the Admiralty hospital and out to the regiments shed light on the kinds of medical drugs being officially provided to the Russian army and navy in the mid-eighteenth century. Chemical medicines are visible, notably the regular inclusion of mercury, but also sal ammoniac, sulphur, vitriol, and antimony.[87] Other official records tell us more about the place of chemical medicine in eighteenth-century Russian military medicine. The 1720 Naval Statute laid down a list of medical supplies that should be kept on all Russian naval vessels: this includes antimony, arsenic, and several mercury compounds.[88] Not only was mercury now an accepted part of official medicine, it was a legally required part of naval medicine. Military medicine, like court medicine and medical books for lay audiences, was increasingly chemically inclined by the early eighteenth century.

From the 1690s to the 1750s we find both a wider variety of chemicals, and much greater evidence of the presence of chemicals in texts and prescriptions, than we did in most of the seventeenth century. Medical books for the tsar, for the Russian elite outside the immediate courtly circles, and for ordinary Muscovites all include chemicals and some even directly announce their chemical medical affiliation. Lists of medicines kept by the Medical Chancellery, and lists of required medicines set out in military regulations, also prominently include chemical medicines, including the mercury that was so hard to track down in seventeenth-century documents. These changes can be directly linked to the foreign medical practitioners of the Apothecary Chancery. Although we see other figures involved along the way, the work of Gurchin and Blumentrost to promote chemical medicine to key patrons and lay audiences from the 1690s on paved the way for a broader acceptance of those medicines in the eighteenth century. The insistence by certain foreign medical practitioners that chemical medicines were appropriate and valuable finally paid off.

CONCLUSION

What can you achieve in a century? If you are an early modern medical practitioner, you can convince the Russian court that chemicals are a legitimate kind of medicine. Before the 1650s, traces of chemicals in official Russian medicine were negligible, and there was some attempt to stop their usage all together. While multiple medical practitioners at the court were pro-chemical medicine, the anti-chemical stance came primarily from Russian officials, informed by their concerns over poisoning. In the second half of the century, medical practitioners directly addressed their patrons and achieved a much greater acceptance of chemical medicines, which then became a regular part of prescriptions in the late seventeenth and early eighteenth century, though, as always, taking up less space than plants. The story of chemicals in seventeenth-century Russian medicine is the story of a rise from insignificance to acceptance.

The rise of chemicals is also, in its way, a global story. This is not the global story of the American medicinal plants; it is not clear where the chemicals came from. Rather, it is a globality of rule creation and negotiation. Raj has shown how co-construction of knowledge was a vital part of the interactions of South Asia and Europe in the early modern period. In early modern Russia, there was a co-construction of rules. Ideas and practices came in from Western Europe, were promoted locally by Western European practitioners, but had to contend with the ideas of Russian bureaucrats and the Russian elite. The Western European practitioners and the Russian officials occupied the same geography, but the ideas they expressed were brought together in the single location of the Apothecary Chancery because of the international links of the court. In the case of chemical medicine, this local exchange created by international links led to a complex, century-long negotiation over the suitability of one kind of *materia medica*.

This negotiation did not take place explicitly. There is no extant document recording an exchange between foreign medical practitioners and Russian administrators setting out their opposing stances on chemical medicine. Rather, we can trace this negotiation through a variety of documents. We can see that medical practitioners like Dee, Gurchin, Guttmensch, and Blumentrost all used chemical medicine, and sometimes went as far as directly promoting it. We can see that Russian officials explicitly banned chemicals in the 1640s oath, and later disregarded the importance of chemical medicine in incidents like the 1690 Padua report. These documents show the push and pull between what medical practitioners wanted to do, and what officials would allow. This push and pull was how the Apothecary Chancery, a hybrid institution combining elements of both Western European and Muscovite practices, created its rules, regulations, and norms of practice. Following chemicals in Muscovy shows how knowledge and rules were co-constructed by diverse actors in the early modern world.

4

The Problems of the Flesh

A key part of medical drugs is their consumption by patients, linking *materia medica* to bodies. This connection represents the value of medical drugs but also the major cause for concern. Throughout the history of the consumption of materials for medical purposes, individuals have fretted about how materials impact bodies. As we saw earlier, people were often concerned about the difference between materials that could heal and materials that could kill. One concern in the early modern world was that the properties of commodities were determined by the region from which they originated and would pass on those qualities to the body that consumed them.[1] This concern that materials would change bodies in undesirable ways sometimes shaped what materials were taken up. Londa Schiebinger has written about agnotology, culturally created ignorance, in the case of the "peacock flower," an abortifacient widely used in the early modern West Indies but rejected by Europeans despite their general enthusiasm for other plants from the Americas.[2] Humans have long worried about what *materia medica* do to their bodies and shaped their consumption habits around them.

Such concerns were hugely important, but they were not monolithic or static. Looking at the histories of medical drugs, food, and spices, we can find numerous examples of how novel substances were incorporated into and even changed a society that initially distrusted them. Non-European consumable goods such as coffee were initially viewed with some skepticism yet over time became accepted and even embraced by European society.[3] Samir Boumedienne, writing of the European appropriation of American *materia medica,* has argued for the "colonisation of knowledge," where knowledge of these American drugs was Europeanized and claimed by Europe, all the better to make those items consumable by Europeans.[4] Marcy Norton has shown that when tobacco and chocolate were brought to Europe they were in some ways adjusted to enter European society but also led to changes in that society.[5] The relationship between the consumer and the consumed was always fraught, but it was also movable.

We find just such a fraught but movable relationship in early modern Russia regarding flesh-based medicines. There were a number of fleshy ingredients, or ingredients extracted from flesh, used in early modern medicine. One example is musk, extracted from the glands of a slaughtered musk deer and commonly used in medicines in the Islamic world and Western Europe.[6] A widespread medicine based on flesh was theriac, a compound drug the creation of which involved transforming the key ingredient of viper's flesh, then thought to be poisonous, into a beneficial medicament.[7] This recipe originated in the ancient Middle East and can be found in medieval and early modern Western European, Islamic, Chinese, Japanese, and Tibetan texts.[8] Early modern medicine even used human flesh. Mumia, part of a category of medicines known as "corpse medicine," was a powder most commonly created from desiccated human flesh from ancient Egyptian mummies, another African *materia medica* in vogue in Western Europe.[9] Flesh-based medicines were a major part of treatments in the early modern global world, yet Russian documents show a distinct reluctance with regards to this specific category of *materia medica.*

The Apothecary Chancery oath of the 1620s names and bans two flesh-based medicines in particular, theriac and mumia, as well as restricting the use of flesh from creatures considered to be poisonous.[10] From the late sixteenth to the mid-seventeenth century Western Europeans, both medics and travellers, commented on this Muscovite concern over flesh-based medicines. From the late sixteenth century on, such foreigners' accounts note that Russians were reluctant to take certain medications, especially on fast days. These accounts also tell us that certain medicines were banned for the whole year and not just on fast days, and it is flesh-based medicines in particular that Western Europeans noted that Russians had specific concerns about. Absences in the Russian prescription records also support the idea that in the sixteenth to mid-seventeenth century Muscovites did not accept flesh-based medicines, in particular theriac and mumia.

We can see here a similar kind of cultural bias to that discussed by Schiebinger. Muscovites generally valued consumable medicines, including those from other traditions and containing ingredients sourced far from the Russian Empire. Indeed, geography also seems to have been unimportant here: mumia in general was banned, without reference to its most common incarnation as an African object or its later history as a product that could be produced anywhere; the flesh of animals native to multiple regions was also banned. This was not an issue of geography, but rather of category. There was a Muscovite agnotology of flesh-based medicines, a culturally constructed rejection and ignorance of that group of medicaments coexisting with the general enthusiasm for consumable medicines as a whole.

The Muscovite agnotology of flesh-based medicines was fundamentally shaped by religion. The early modern Russian Orthodox Church, the dominant religion of the empire, had very strict rules about the behaviour of humans, including the foods and drinks they could consume, rules directly referenced by the Western Europeans writing about Muscovite restrictions and bans on flesh-based medicines. There were also strict rules about the treatment of dead bodies in Muscovy. Although saints' bodies elsewhere in the Christian world could be separated into parts, Muscovite saints were kept whole. Post-mortem examinations were rarely performed in early modern Russia, and when they were, the act of cutting into the body was unusual, and such examinations vociferously protested as a violation. Both theriac and mumia violated Russian Orthodox Christian rules on consumption; mumia also violated the rules on the proper treatment of dead bodies. The agnotology of flesh-based medicines then was an issue of the correct treatment of the Muscovite Christian body.

This agnotology did not last. By the late seventeenth century, there was some limited mention of theriac and, to a lesser extent, mumia in medical records. Both are present in the eighteenth-century records. Even more interestingly, a key adviser of Peter the Great, Stefan Iavorskii, wrote sermons in the early eighteenth century using theriac as a positive metaphor. This shift from rejection to acceptance of flesh-based medicines took place during two other major changes regarding Russian thought on dead bodies. The Russian Orthodox Church under Peter the Great cracked down on unofficial saints' cults, which often involved the veneration of dead bodies, and Peter the Great also opened the Kunstkamera, a museum the Russian public was encouraged to visit that prominently featured anatomical specimens. We can see the history of flesh-based medicines in early modern Russia as a history of the construction and destruction of an agnotology regarding objects both local and global.

THE MUSCOVITE BODY

Ideas about the human body were fundamental to the issue of flesh-based medicines in early modern Russia.[11] The Russian Empire was multi-ethnic and multi-religious, but ruled and dominated by members of the Russian Orthodox Church, and it was the teachings of that church that underpinned Muscovite responses to flesh-based medicines. Those teachings covered, among other things, sacred time, laws of consumption, and rites of burial. A major kind of sacred time for the Russian Orthodox Christian Church was fast days, when the kinds of objects suitable for consumption by a Russian Orthodox Christian were closely restricted. Those restrictions of fast days were themselves a sub-set of broader laws of consumption that continuously regulated what a Russian Orthodox Christian should and should not eat or drink. Once dead, concerns shifted to how the body itself was treated. To understand how the Muscovite agnotology of flesh-based medicines was created, we need to begin with religious thought on human bodies.

The sacred time of fast days was a particular kind of restriction over consumption. According to Julia Herzberg, "Fast days made up 180 to 220 days of the Orthodox church year," or up to 60 per cent of the calendar year.[12] Fasts then substantially affected what Muscovites could eat and drink throughout the year. Those restrictions primarily limited the consumption of dairy and meat.[13] The restrictions were taken seriously, including by the royal family. Tsar Aleksei Mikhailovich maintained his own strict fasting rules and imposed them on others. Other major figures of seventeenth century Russia were also keen on the strict maintenance of the fasting regime. Unsurprisingly, the notoriously strict Schismatic churchman Avvakum Petrov, who would later become a kind of figurehead to the Old Believer movement, also carefully observed fasts and insisted that others should as well.[14] Moreover, Avvakum saw disease as punishment for sin and repentance, and viewed proper religious observance – including observing fasts – as the only road to healing.[15] The stringent rules for fasting that limited the consumption of animal products on fast days were carefully applied during the sixteenth and seventeenth centuries and religious concepts of illness, healing, and the correct state of the body were fundamental to Muscovite life.

According to foreign visitors to Russia, those rules affected not only which foods could be eaten but also which medicines could be taken. The British diplomat Giles Fletcher, writing of his time in Russia in the late 1580s, said:

> They [the Russians] make a difference of meats and drinks, accounting the use of one to be more holy than of another. And therefore in their set fasts they forbear to eat flesh and white meats (as we call them) after the manner of the popish superstition [Catholicism], which they observe so strictly and with such blind devotion as that they will rather die than eat one bit of flesh, eggs, or such like, for the health of their bodies in their extreme sickness.[16]

Fletcher, then, tells us that Russians of the 1580s would restrict the contents of their consumable medicines due to fast-day restrictions in particular on the consumption of certain kinds of flesh. Moreover, he states that this adherence to fast rules was considered more important than medical exigency, that a Russian would refuse life-saving medical treatment rather than break a fast.

Nearly a century later, the British physician Samuel Collins echoed Fletcher's comments about the impact of fast days on medicine in his work *The Present State of Russia*, which recounts his experiences in 1660s Moscow. Collins states: "If a Medicine has *Cor. Cervi* [deer horn], *ungul. Al.* [moose hoof] or *pil. lepor.* [hares' hair] in it, they [Russians] will not take it, though to save their lives, so precise are they in observing their Fasts."[17] Again, we see a foreign observer noting how fast days impacted the consumption of medicines, particularly flesh-based medicines, to the extent that a Muscovite would risk death rather than contravene fasting rules. Importantly, Collins was actually employed by the Apothecary Chancery, so he had direct experience of what could and could not be prescribed to the Russian elite. This intersection of fasting rules with *materia medica* was a key limitation on the practice of medical drugs in Russia, as has been noted by the historian of medicine Sabine Dumschat as well as the food historian Julia Herzberg.[18] Rules of fasting were more important to Muscovites than secular medical guidance.

Russian Orthodox Christians also followed rules regarding what could be consumed on non-fast days: they consumed the host, communion wine, and drank holy water, all sanctified objects appropriate to, and so beneficial for, the human body. Conversely, even on non-fast days certain foods were banned, restrictions that particularly affected what kinds of meat could be eaten. One such kind of meat was turtle meat. Julia Herzberg recounts a dramatic violation of this rule in the early eighteenth century, when Peter the Great fed some guests turtle meat without their knowledge. Several guests, being shown the shells from which this meat had been taken, were then violently ill.[19] Other than showing Peter the Great's disdain for the Russian Orthodox Christian rules of consumption that his father Aleksei Mikhailovich had so carefully upheld, this incident is telling about the reactions of devout Russian Orthodox Christians to breaches of fasting rules. His guests were horrified, even to the point of physical illness, to have inadvertently broken the rules. Restrictions and bans on the consumption of meat were serious, and violations a major incident.

Although Collins complained about how the Russian Orthodox Church's consumption rules affected prescribing practices, there was some shared ground between Russian Orthodox Christian and Western European medical views of the human body. Despite the rise of chemical medicine during this period, humoralism remained a key idea in understanding human bodies into the eighteenth century. The rebalancing of the humours central to this kind of medicine could involve removing a substance from the body, such as by bleeding, but often involved consuming specific materials or refraining to consume others depending on your specific humoral makeup. This is not so different from Muscovites' religious behaviour in which consuming certain materials – such as communion wine – is good for the body, whereas others – like turtle meat – are bad. Pre-modern medical and religious figures alike saw consumption as a major way to maintain the correct state of the human body, and so both aimed to strictly control that consumption, albeit sometimes in ways that directly contradicted each other.

The state of the human body seen as the ideal could differ, particularly when it came to male bodies. Early modern medicine and early modern Russian Orthodox Christianity shared similar views on what constituted an ideal female body: one that could bear children.[20] In contrast, sixteenth-century Muscovite icons typically depicted male saints with emaciated bodies, with the image emphasizing visible rib bones and thin cheeks, showing that the saint kept strictly to both religious rules of consumption and the norm of asceticism expected of religious figures. By the late seventeenth century this began to change, and icons started to portray bodies that were less gaunt. Avvakum Petrov strongly opposed this development. For Avvakum, an emaciated body was a correctly religious body, showing that the inhabitant was eating only enough to stay alive and certainly keeping strictly within the rules of consumption set out by Russian Orthodox Christianity.[21] Such an approach fundamentally clashed with medical aims to maintain a body in the peak of health.

After death the human body continued to be subject to strict religious rules. Muscovite bodies were promptly buried in a Christian ritual without being embalmed, sometimes as soon as twenty-four hours after, unless they had died in the winter in which case they had to be left in a charnel house until the earth thawed.[22] One folk prayer against alcohol consumption called for using an exhumed human corpse as a part of the ritual, but as a rule Muscovites did not exhume the dead.[23] Post-mortem examinations were rare in Muscovy, and typically involved an external examination rather than an autopsy proper; only one record of a case that involved cutting into the body survives.[24] All such post-mortems were unpopular, and the clerk responsible for their organization was given the nickname "seller of the dead" [*mertvoprodavets*].[25] The correct treatment of the Russian Orthodox Christian body was to bury it intact and unaltered as soon as possible after death in accordance with Christian practice, and to leave the body in its grave.

These practices would have been broadly familiar to Western European Christians, but there was one area of dealing with corpses where Russian Orthodox and Western European branches of Christianity notably differed: the treatment of saints' bodies. Both Catholicism and Russian Orthodox Christianity believed in the existence of saints and the role their bodies played in Christianity, including faith healing; the Protestant churches rejected such practices.[26] Where Russian Orthodox Christianity and Catholicism differed was in how the saints' bodies should be treated. As Katherine Park has shown, the Latin church allowed for saints' bodies to be divided into discrete parts to increase the number of relics, all of which could then be venerated.[27] In contrast, Gail Lenhoff has established that there was a focus in pre-modern Russia on the saintly corpse remaining intact.[28] The resistance to post-mortems, the lack of embalming, and the insistence on the completeness of saints' bodies demonstrate that for Muscovites, the correct treatment of all dead bodies was to lay them to rest complete, intact, and unmodified.

Considering fasts, laws on consumption, and rules for burial, we can build a picture of Russian Orthodox Christian views on the correct treatment of human bodies. The condition of the human body was a statement of that person's commitment to God, and following strict rules of consumption – even to the point of emaciation – was a proclamation of that commitment. Rules limiting consumption primarily applied to animal products, including meat, making the consumption of some kinds of flesh conditional on the rhythms of sacred and mundane time, and of other kinds of flesh entirely taboo. Those rules were so important that Russians would rather follow them and be ill than break them and be treated. Rules concerning the correct treatment of bodies extended after death, with corpses being swiftly buried intact. These rules limited what flesh a human body could consume, and how the fleshy human body could be treated, both of which substantially impacted Muscovy's attitude to early modern medicine's use of flesh-based medicines.

PROBLEMATIC CORPSES

Muscovites had very specific ideas about how living humans should behave, and how dead humans should be treated. These two points converged in official approaches to corpse medicine. The Apothecary Chancery oath of the late 1620s banned medical staff from prescribing "unclean mumia," referring to a powder created from the desiccated flesh of human corpses.[29] Other Apothecary Chancery documents from the first half of the seventeenth century indicate that this ban was enforced. Here, we need to examine the global history of mumia, what it was, where it came from, and what role it came to play in Western European medicine, and we need to look at Russian documents dealing with corpse medicine. All of this is necessary to understand why the Western European practitioners at the Moscow court might have wanted to prescribe this medicine, and why Russian officials in the first half of the seventeenth century did not let them.

By the time of the Apothecary Chancery oath of the 1620s, mumia, also known as mumie or mummy, had been around for some time.[30] How exactly early modern medicine came to use powdered corpse has to do with the transmission of ancient world medical ideas, the specific history of which in the case of mumia has been outlined by Karl Dannenfeldt. Dannenfeldt tells us that

> by the time of the Renaissance mummy had become a highly prized drug. In medical tradition pissasphalt from the near east had long

> been recognized as a curative drug. In trade it was usually called *mumia*. Since the appearance of this natural pissasphalt was similar to that of the bituminous materials used by the ancient Egyptians in the mummification process, it became the practice to substitute the materials found in the bodies of the Egyptian mummies for the natural product. Abd Allatif, the Arabian historian and physician, writing in Cairo in 1203, remarks, "The mummy found in the hollows of corpses in Egypt, differs but immaterially from the nature of mineral mummy; and where any difficulty arises in procuring the latter, may be substituted in its stead." The next step was to substitute the dried flesh of the mummy for the hardened bituminous deposits found in the cavities of bodies.[31]

This conflation of a mineral from the Middle East with the preserved flesh of mummified bodies from North Africa led to the use of powdered desiccated human flesh in early modern Western European medicine.[32] By the time the Russian court was first recruiting foreign medical practitioners, the use of this human corpse powder was well established in Western Europe.

The origins of mumia are linked to ancient North African mummified corpses; some Western European medical thinkers came to believe that rather more recent and local corpses could also be used for mumia.[33] Paracelsus recommended the use of the "body of a person who dies an unnatural rather than a natural death, before falling ill," and that a corpse should only be left for a day and a night before the mumia was created. According to Katherine Park, Paracelsus also gives practical thought to where to obtain such fresh corpses: those of executed criminals would do nicely.[34] In 1609 Paracelsus's follower Oswald Crollius gave a longer account on how to make this mumia from fresh corpses: "the carcass of a red-haired man twenty-four years old, who had been hanged, broken on the wheel, or thrust-through, exposed to the air for a day and a night, then cut into small pieces or slices, sprinkled with a little powder of myrrh and aloes, soaked in spirits of wine, dried, soaked again, and dried."[35] The mumia the Apothecary Chancery banned could have been that of ancient North African or more recent European corpses.

Indeed, as much as mumia was a particular kind of medicament, it was also a medicament associated with a specific geography. Although today we use the word "mummy" to mean preserved corpses in general, at the start of this period it referred only to those Egyptian preserved corpses Abd Allatif recommended as a substitute for a Middle Eastern mineral. This particular association of preserved corpses, the Middle East, and North Africa shows up elsewhere in pre-modern Afro-Eurasia: the sixteenth-century Chinese medical author Li Shenzhen wrote of a "honey mummy" he had heard of from Islamic sources as being created in Arabia.[36] The writings of Paracelsus and Crollius in the late sixteenth and early seventeenth centuries began to reframe "mumia" in Europe as potentially European, but mummies primarily remained a product of the Middle East and North Africa. It took Spanish engagement with South American preserved bodies over the same period to begin to gradually shift the meaning of that term towards the broader present-day sense of any preserved corpse.[37] Yet we should be cautious to abandon the specific geography of mumia and of mummies too quickly. Paracelsus's trick was something he created in response to the use of North African corpses, a gruesome counterpart to the medical practitioners who sought to replace American botanicals with local plants.[38] Mumia was first of all a product of the Middle East and North Africa that had a global history in texts and practices across Afro-Eurasia.

Yet not all mumia was human flesh, North African or otherwise. In the eighteenth century Samuel Johnson wrote that "we have two different substances preserved for medical use under the name of mummy; one is the dried flesh of human bodies embalmed with myrrh and spices; the other is the liquor running from such mummies when newly prepared, or when affected by great heat, or by damps."[39] Mumia could be powdered, desiccated human flesh, a liquid exuded by a corpse, or the original minerals meant in ancient world texts. In each case, the medicament was still a global product, involving the use of spices from Asia and myrrh from East Africa. When relying solely on the presence of the word "mumia" we cannot be sure of the precise nature of the object described. Here, we can turn back to the phrasing of the Apothecary Chancery oath, which describes mumia as "unclean," *nechistii*, meaning unclean in a ritual sense.[40] It is unlikely that pissasphalt or bitumen would have aroused such strong language. Given the strict rules over the consumption of flesh in early modern Russia, when the Apothecary Chancery banned mumia, they were most likely banning a substance created from human flesh, whether European or African.

We can trace the Apothecary Chancery's disapproval of mumia beyond the ban in the 1620s oath. None of the five extant import lists from the first half of the seventeenth century mention mumia, nor do any of the thirty-four extant prescriptions created between 1629 and 1645.[41] Absences are always tricky. We know more prescriptions were written than survived, and so there could be lost prescriptions that do list the substance. Although Egyptian mumia would have had to have been imported, it would be possible for a Paracelsian working in the Apothecary Chancery to create the fresh kind of mumia proposed by Paracelsus in Moscow, which would then not appear in import records but would in prescriptions. Yet if mumia was in regular use in the department in this period we would expect to find at least some trace of it in the surviving documents. The absence of mumia from import lists and prescriptions of the 1620s–1640s cannot definitively determine that it was not used by the Apothecary Chancery, but it does indicate that it was not a regular part of official medicine in this period.

Other sources indicate that there was some corpse medicine being used in unofficial Russian medicine in the early seventeenth century. Martinus Bäer, a German Lutheran pastor resident in Moscow from 1600 to 1612 who had close links to the Russian court, wrote in his *Chronicle of Muscovy* [*Chronicon Muscoviticum*, translated into Russian as *Letopis Moskovskaia*]:

> The devilish massacre lasted from 3 o'clock to 11 [o'clock]. 2135 Poles were killed; Among those killed were students, German jewellers and merchants of Augsburg, who had a lot of money and other kinds of goods. The villains threw the bodies of the murdered into the streets as ą sacrifice to dogs and local Russian medical practitioners [lit: Russian town-square healers], who cut fat from the corpses. For two days they lay dead on the street [lit: under the open sky]; on the third day, the killer Shuisky ordered them to be picked up and buried in God's house [equivalent to Potter's field].[42]

This is not a description of the creation of mumia, but rather the use of human fat, which was also used in early modern European medicine to make a kind of salve, with executioners often supplying, and sometimes also applying, this product of their trade.[43] The local doctors mentioned here were making just such a salve.

Interesting here is how this human-fat-based medicine is presented. Bäer clearly views this as an inappropriate practice and – significantly for our purposes – a violation of the correct Christian burial rites we saw above, as he specifically notes that the corpses were left outside for days and allowed to be mauled before finally being taken for Christian burial. Also important is when this incident occurred. Bäer dates these events to 1606, during a dynastic crisis known as the Time of Troubles (1598–1613). His mention of "the killer Shuisky" is a reference to Vasilii Shuisky and his ousting and killing of the First False Dmitrii after the latter had taken the Russian throne under the pretence of being the youngest son of Ivan the Terrible (who had in fact died in 1591).[44] The nineteenth-century historian L.F. Zmeev repeats this corpse medicine incident in a mangled fashion, temporally relocating it to the occupation of Moscow by Polish forces in 1610–11, which was also a particularly violent period of the Time of Troubles with armed uprisings against the Poles. Zmeev also edits Bäer's account, calling them just "town-square healers" and juxtaposing this with a comment on the popularity of such corpse medicine with certain of the foreign medics.[45] Those edits both serve to distance Russians from this practice, even as Bäer specifically accuses them. Both Bäer and Zmeev then, despite the differences in their accounts, associate this corpse medicine not only with a tumultuous period, but with specific violent events.

By including this description of corpse medicine, Bäer takes part in a trend in contemporary depictions of the Time of Troubles. One tale, the dramatically titled *Bewailing of Captivity* [*Plach' o plenenii*], describes the Time of Troubles as follows: "[Russia] which previously was so brilliant, like the morning star, fell from highest heaven."[46] The historians N.V. Rybalko and D.V. Liseitsev have done much to reframe the Time of Troubles as a more mundane and everyday place than that described in the vivid colours and emotive rhetoric of works like the *Bewailing of Captivity*.[47] Bäer's tale of flagrant corpse robbers in the very centre of Moscow has more in common with the florid, emotive prose of the *Bewailing of Captivity* than it does with the sober bureaucratic texts that Liseitsev and Rybalko have brought to light. Indeed, the pointed inclusion of this incident in the *Chronicle of Muscovy* might even be read as a rhetorical device, inserting into a narrative of the Time of Troubles what many saw as an evil practice – the use of human corpses in medicine – as a medical measure of Bäer's horror at the events of the Time of Troubles. Yet again, figures associated with the Russian court in the early seventeenth century saw corpse medicine as a fundamentally, almost iconically, bad practice.

The 1620s Apothecary Chancery oath was then created by a confluence of events not only within the Russian Empire but also across the Middle East, North Africa, and Western Eurasia from the ancient period up until the early seventeenth century. Ancient world texts from the Middle East recommending kinds of minerals were misinterpreted as recommending desiccated human flesh, which was incorporated into the Western European medicine from which Russia took so much of its official medicine. Although there was an unofficial practice of corpse medicine in Russia, this was strongly disapproved by the Moscow court based on Russian Orthodox Christian ideas on the consumption of flesh and the treatment of dead bodies, and the Apothecary Chancery did not use such corpse medicine in the early seventeenth century. Corpse medicine was available to Muscovites because of the international links of the court, but it was local religious practices that led to the early seventeenth-century agnotology at the court regarding this kind of medicine.

EVIL SNAKES

Mumia was not the only Western European flesh-based medicine to which the Russians took exception in the early seventeenth century. Returning to the Apothecary Chancery oath of the late 1620s, alongside "unclean mumia" we also see an imprecation not to use "any evil snake poison nor other poisonous animal nor reptile nor bird."[48] As well as desiccated human flesh, the Apothecary Chancery was restricting other kinds of fleshy medicines. In part, this returns us to the general Russian Orthodox rules restricting the consumption of all kinds of meat on fast days, and some kinds of meat on all days. It also again shows us how those Russian Orthodox rules significantly intersected with the trajectory of specific medicaments in official Russian medicine. In early seventeenth-century Russia there was an agnotology not only of corpse medicine, but of flesh-based medicines more broadly.

We can trace this issue of animal-based medicines conflicting with Russian Orthodox rules of consumption in foreign accounts as well. In the 1600s Jacques Margeret, a French traveller to Muscovy, wrote:

> They do not know of medical practitioners, except the Emperor and some major Lords. They hold several things to be dirty, which are used in Medicine, among other things they will not gladly take pills.

> As for Clysters, they abhor them, along with Musk, Civet, and other such things. But if the simple [people] are sick, they take a good dosing of acqua vitae, and will add to it arquebouze powder, or a piece of crushed garlic, stir it and drink, and go that moment to a bathhouse, which is so hot that we almost could not endure it, but they remain there until they have sweated for an hour or even two, and they do the same for every disease.[49]

Like Fletcher, Margeret also viewed Russians as being particularly cautious in their use of *materia medica.*

The specific medical items and processes Margeret mentions are also significant. He notes that musk, the product of an animal native to Asia but in the early modern world seen as originating in Tibet specifically, was "abhorred" in Muscovy.[50] Also scorned was civet, most likely civet musk, the glandular secretion from that cat species which is mostly found in sub-Saharan Africa and South Asia. Two of the items mentioned by Margeret were then flesh-based medicines created by the products of animals native to Africa and Asia. He also informs us of a dislike of pills, which could contain a range of ingredients, as well as clysters, an early modern term for an enema. Margeret's list of the Muscovites' specific dislikes then covers processes like clysters, but, as with other foreign accounts from this period, he makes specific note of the dislike of flesh-based global medicines.

Margeret's account broadly coincides with that of the Apothecary Chancery oath in the restrictions of certain flesh-based medicines. We find greater overlap with the oath if we return to the British physician Samuel Collins. Collins continued his ruminations on the medical habits of Muscovites by saying

> That which is *Pogano* (or unclean) many not be eaten at anytime; as Horse flesh, Mares-milk, Asses-milk, Hares, Squirrels, Coneys [rabbits], Elks: *Theriaca* or Treacle,[51] is *Pogano* because it has Vipers flesh in it. *Castorium* [Beaver bile], Musk, and Civet are not to be used internally amongst them. Sugar-Candy, and Loaf-Sugar are *Scarumni,* or prohibited in Fasting-dayes; a Knife that has cut Flesh is *Scarumna* for a *Sootky,* or twenty four hours.[52]

Here, Collins's mention of *Theriaca,* and his note that it contains vipers' flesh, is key. The Apothecary Chancery oath uses the phrase evil snake poison, which is a reference to viper's flesh, then thought to be poisonous, yet a key ingredient in the highly valued medicament theriac. Collins underlines that the Russian dislike of theriac was based specifically on the presence in that medicine of viper's flesh. Both the Apothecary Chancery oath and several foreign sources note a general distrust of flesh-based medicines at the early seventeenth-century Russian court; Collins and the oath specifically point us towards the medicine theriac and its key ingredient of viper's flesh as a major point of concern.

As with mumia, other Apothecary Chancery documents support the idea of a restriction on the use of theriac in the early seventeenth century. Of the twenty-four extant prescriptions from 1629 to 1645, none of them mention theriac or viper's flesh.[53] Similarly, the three extant import lists from the first half of the seventeenth century also do not list those items.[54] Yet one term does complicate this picture: scorpion oil, which appears in one prescription and two import lists.[55] There were two medicaments that were referred to by this name during the early modern period. One is, unsurprisingly, created by frying scorpions in olive oil, recommended in a number of texts from the medieval period on.[56] The other was invented in the sixteenth century by the Italian physician Pietro Andrea Mattioli and was created from 123 ingredients, combining the ingredients of theriac with that of the related medicine mithradatum. In fact, Mattioli's scorpion oil was referred to by contemporaries as "a liquid theriac."[57] Without further details – which these documents do not provide – it is unclear which of these two scorpion oils is meant in the Russian documents. Theriac *qua* theriac was neither imported nor prescribed during the first half of the seventeenth century, but it could have had a limited presence there undercover as scorpion oil.

To better understand the Apothecary Chancery's objections to theriac, we need to turn to the history of that medicine. Theriac – an ancient world compound made from many ingredients, including the viper's flesh then thought poisonous – was famous across the pre-modern world. An early detailed recipe was written by Nicander of Colophon ca 200 BCE.[58] By the eleventh century it was mentioned, under the name *tiryaq*, in the Islamic pharmacopoeia of al-Biruni, and theriac is also found in early modern Chinese, Japanese, and Tibetan texts.[59] It was long popular in Western Europe: in sixteenth-century Venice, correct preparation of theriac was an officially regulated and observed process; it was listed in German and French official pharmacopoeias into the late nineteenth century.[60] Theriac was considered a valuable medicine across much of pre-modern Eurasia, yet not in the Apothecary Chancery in the early seventeenth century.

The Apothecary Chancery's objections to theriac were partly based on the religious restrictions on the consumption of flesh. Yet there was also another reason, related to what Western Europeans saw as the virtues of theriac. How exactly theriac did what it did, how the workings of this extraordinary medicine should be understood philosophically, was the subject of serious intellectual work and much debate in the ancient Mediterranean world, the Islamic and Latin Christian medieval worlds, and early modern Western Europe and China. As Carla Nappi has argued, "Over the course of its global history, theriac was both poison and antidote."[61] Indeed, even those who praised its virtues were not always in agreement as to *how* it worked. Originally, theriac was developed to treat snakebites. Here, the issue was sympathy: the poison of the viper's flesh acted in sympathy to the poison in the bite, and so neutralized it. By the medieval period it was used as an antidote to poison more generally, and was in common use against the plague, a disease viewed as akin to poison.[62] These specific uses eventually faded away, and by the early modern period a medicine once meant to sympathetically counteract poison was seen as a panacea and used to treat almost any disease.

Key to debates over the nature and uses of the drug was theriac's status as a compound medicine.[63] It was not always understood as such: Chinese texts classified it as an animal-based simple.[64] But in Western Eurasia – whence the Russian court took their understanding of it – theriac was a compound. A number of thinkers focused on this in understanding its action, with William of Brescia saying that its virtue was due to the properties it received in fermentation when ingredients were combined through pharmaceutical methods; in this he followed both Ibn Sina and Galen.[65] According to this logic, the nature of the *ingredients* of theriac – the poisonous viper's flesh included – would be transformed through slow and complicated pharmaceutical processes into the virtues of the *drug* theriac. Theriac was, in the most literal sense, greater than the sum of its parts.

In contrast to William of Brescia and others' thoughts on the differences between the properties of ingredients and the properties of the drug, in the 1620s Apothecary Chancery oath a very direct and simplistic line is drawn between medicament and effect: viper's flesh is poison;

medicine made from it must have a negative effect on the human body. Such a direct line of thinking is also evident in other seventeenth-century Russian documents about healing. One example comes from a witchcraft case from 1657, in which the accused, one Andrei Durbenev, defended his possession of herbs, stating: "One root is taken by people for stomach complaints [lit. womb] and for difficulty breathing, and the second root is for horses, it is given to broken-winded horses,[66] and the third root is for teeth, it grows in fields and kitchen gardens."[67] Here Durbenev draws a straight line between medicament and effect: the sufferer is to take one herb, and it will have an effect. A similar line of reasoning is found in a seventeenth-century medical book: "There is an herb called 'bronets,' which grows in bushes, like peas, the colour of a crow, blue berries. And that herb is good. If a person has an old wound or an old hernia, then take that herb and mix it with honey, and that [medicine] will drive any unclean thing from the body, and make the eyes bright, and prevent coughs."[68] Here, again, there is a single herb, which is good, and it will affect the body in a direct and positive way.

Such medicines stand in direct contrast to theriac, composed of forty ingredients, at least one of which – viper's flesh – was considered essentially bad, and created using complex procedures over months, resulting in a transformation of the ingredients. The Apothecary Chancery oaths followed a similar logic to these simple remedies: ingredients relate directly to the effect of a medicine, and so if an ingredient is bad, the medicine must also be bad. Theriac was thus rejected by the Russian court in the early seventeenth century as the inclusion of poisonous snake flesh in it was not compatible with the idea of a simple, direct relationship between medical ingredients and the effect on the human body, which was how they understood *materia medica*. The early seventeenth-century agnotology of flesh-based medicines in Russia was then based partly on religious considerations, and partly on ideas on how *materia medica* functioned.

THERIAC REHABILITATED

In the 1620s, the Apothecary Chancery denounced theriac, that ancient Middle Eastern snakebite remedy reconceptualized by early modern Western Europeans as a trusted panacea, as "evil snake poison." Yet by the 1680s theriac would be in some use in official medicines; by the 1730s it was regularly included in the medicines sent to the Russian army.

In the early eighteenth century it even became accepted enough to be used as a positive metaphor in speeches. This was a remarkable and dramatic reversal of opinion on a major medicament, and, crucially, it came about during massive social and cultural change that affected how Russians viewed consumables.

Theriac started to appear irregularly in official Russian medical records in the late seventeenth century. It was certainly prescribed by 1664, as in December of that year the Apothecary Chancery twice prescribed *Fir'iaku vinitseiskogo*, Venetian theriac, to a Kalmyk emissary.[69] In 1671, the department prescribed theriaca andromachi, a common variant of theriac that typically included viper's flesh.[70] Theriac was related to the compound medicine mithradatum, and the Apothecary Chancery also prescribed that medicine at least once, in 1675.[71] Theriaca andromachi appears again later in the century, in a purchase list from 1679 and a prescription from 1698.[72] These documents do not tell us the ingredients of either the theriaca andromachi or the mithradatum. Although these are names attached to established recipes, substitutions and falsifications could and did happen; we can never be entirely confident about the precise ingredients of such compounds in any particular instance based on the name alone. However, we can make reasonable presumptions by looking at what was typically found in compounds going under those names. Based on other sources from Western Europe that do provide us with the various different recipes used for each, the mithradatum is unlikely to have contained viper's flesh, whereas the theriaca andromachi most likely did.[73]

Theriac shows up in the eighteenth-century Medical Chancellery records multiple times. Theriac was sent to the Russian army in October 1736, the very start of documentary preservation for that department.[74] It was sent to the army no less than ten times in 1737, a practice that continued until at least 1750.[75] Alongside the growing official use of theriac from the late seventeenth into the early eighteenth century, medical texts created by Apothecary Chancery staff aimed at a lay audience also show interest in theriac. The royal *Domestic and Field Pharmacy* presented to Peter the Great by Daniel Gurchin and Laurentius Blumentrost senior in 1698 mentions theriac.[76] It was perhaps the first Russian-language medical text to recommend this medicament: neither Gurchin's *Extract from Doctor's Knowledge*, produced only two years earlier, nor his Apothecary Chancery *Pharmacopoeia* of 1676 mention it. A later work that Gurchin is proposed to have authored, the *Small Domestic Pharmacy* [*Aptechka domovaia*], does mentions theriac.[77] Both official medical records and medical books created by official medical practitioners demonstrate a growing acceptance of theriac across the late seventeenth and into the first half of the eighteenth century.

Other Russian-language medical works of this period also mention theriac. The *Little Ark of Medicine* [*Kovchezhets meditsinskii*], translated from an as-yet-unidentified Latin text in or after 1730, mentions two kinds of theriac: the now familiar theriaca andromachi, and also theriaca caelestis.[78] Regarding theriaca caelestis, it tells us:

> No. 76 Theriaca caelestis
> For calming excessively disturbed spirits and humors, alleviating disease, and ameliorating nagging ailments, take 1111 [*sic*] grams in Rhenish [wine] or similar, it is good drunk by itself, or in combination with recipes no. 25, 72, 82, 88.[79]

The *Little Ark of Medicine* does not give us any sense of the ingredients of theriaca caelestis, but rather instructions on when and how to take it. Notably, of the four other recipes readers are encouraged to take alongside theriaca caelestis, one of them, no. 72, was theriaca andromachi.[80] Readers of Russian medical texts in the late seventeenth and early eighteenth centuries were increasingly likely to encounter theriac, and were sometimes even recommended to take more than one kind.

There is some evidence that lay readers of these medical texts would have been able to buy theriac. We can return here to the Dutch trade documents on early eighteenth-century Russian import tariffs.[81] The Dutch documents on the 1731 Russian tariff list theriac as a commodity with a regular tax price.[82] These are not records of actual trade, but rather of what the Russians expected to be imported sufficiently regularly for it to be worthwhile setting a regular tariff price, and, importantly, goods that were not for government use but for sale on the open market. By 1731, a century after Apothecary Chancery staff were made to swear never to use that drug, and rather less than a century since Samuel Collins had discussed the Russian dislike for the famous compound, the Russian government expected their trading partners to be regularly importing theriac to Russia for sale on the open market, meaning that readers of the *Small Home Pharmacy* and the *Little Ark of Medicine* could find the theriac those texts recommended.

The Russian army staff being officially prescribed theriac, and the private customers buying Dutch imports of it, may also have heard about that medicament in a rather different context. In 1711, Peter the Great's renowned spin doctor and adviser, Stefan Iavorskii, gave a sermon called *Theriac Made from Poison* [*Theriaca ex venenis confecta*], which uses theriac as a metaphor for finding success in defeat.[83] Iavorskii returned to this topic in 1718, with a sermon entitled *In the Celebrated Royal City of St Petersburg [A Sermon on] the Great Theriac, Fruit of Detrimental Ingredients [Made Into a] Useful and Vital Medicine.* [*In celebrima regia urbe Peterburgenst Theriaca Maximus ex adverstatibus fructus, utilitas et animae medicina*]. Iavorskii found theriac to be useful, at least as a political metaphor.

In the 1711 sermon, Iavorskii acknowledges the poisonous ingredients of theriac and states that there is a Russian name for it, *friak*. The Apothecary Chancery called it *teriak* or *fir'iak*, the second of which is fairly close to the term Iavorskii lists.[84] Significantly, Iavorskii links theriac to his idea of an alchemist God, able to change poison to remedy. Iavorskii gives this a political twist: as God can transform what is unclean to be pure, or change a poisonous snake into the marvellous theriac remedy, Peter the Great can change a bitter failure into sweet success. According to Robert Collis, he likely meant here the defeat of the combined Russian and Moldovan armies by the Turks and their Crimean Tatar allies at Pruth in the same year.[85] Iavorskii valued theriac as a metaphor precisely because of its reputation as a drug created by changing poisonous viper's flesh to miraculous cure.

Such an idea is hugely significant to the history of theriac in Russia: it was exactly this aspect of theriac – that poisonous ingredients could be so changed by pharmaceutical production processes that the resulting compound was a famous cure – that led it to be rejected in the 1620s. The transformative aspect of theriac, which was doubted and dismissed by the Russian court in the early seventeenth century, was wholeheartedly accepted by Iavorskii in the 1710s, and promoted by him to the Russian public, who could now not only read about the medicinal value of theriac in their pharmacy texts, take it in their official and unofficial medicines, but also hear about its philosophical value as well.

It is significant that it was specifically Iavorskii who wrote about theriac. Iavorskii was a close confident of Peter the Great, who himself held significant views on the consumption of flesh. In stark contrast to his ascetic father Aleksei Mikhailovich, Peter the Great was against the Russian Orthodox Christian tradition of fasting. During his reign, Peter limited and marginalized the same fasting rules his father had personally upheld and promoted. Peter himself did not fast. Beyond this, he also had little time for general restrictions on certain kinds of consumption. He created and headed the All-Drunken Council, a group of his friends and advisers notorious for its excessive consumption, especially of alcohol.[86] The rehabilitation of theriac occurred at a time when the ruler was advocating and modelling a substantially less restrictive attitude to consumption than had been the case under more religiously observant tsars.

The change in the status of theriac was then linked to changes in Russian culture. It was also linked to changes in Russian medicine. Key here is *change*. The people making and recommending theriac believed one of its central ingredients to be poisonous, yet the final product to not be so, because the elaborate preparations transformed the viper's flesh into something good. This was a logic lost on the Moscow court of the early seventeenth century, when medical ingredients were typically expected to display a direct relationship between the nature of the ingredient, the nature of the final drug, and the effect on the human body. Good ingredients made good medicines which had a good effect on the human body; bad ingredients made bad medicines that had a bad effect.

Over the course of the seventeenth century, the Moscow court came into contact with practices combining and changing ingredients into compound medicines, practices that notably changed the ingredients as a part of the process. Such an approach was heavily promoted by the chemical physicians, who encountered some success in their activities in the late seventeenth century.[87] The rehabilitation of theriac being near-simultaneous to the rise of chemical medicine was not coincidental; the royal *Domestic and Field Pharmacy* contained both a recipe for theriac and Gurchin's dramatic declaration of his allegiance to chemical medicine. All that the Moscow court had learned about pharmaceutical processes and compound remedies, all that the chemical physicians tried so hard to sell over the course of the seventeenth century, directly impacted the reputation of theriac, transforming it in the minds of the Russian elite from a poison to a cure.

Agnotology, in Schiebinger's words, can be "culturally induced ignorances of nature's body."[88] Yet no culture is static. As culture changes, so, then, can agnotologies be created, modified, and destroyed. Early seventeenth-century Russia had an agnotology of flesh-based medicines, including of the logic of how theriac could be a virtuous medicine even though it contained a poisonous ingredient. As Russian culture shifted in the late seventeenth and early eighteenth centuries, including the importance of Russian Orthodox Christian rules of consumption, attitudes to at least some flesh-based medicines also changed. Medical developments fuelled this. As chemical medicine, with its focus on pharmaceutical techniques of creating medicines, began to make a mark on official Russian medicine, views on the transformation central to the creation of theriac did too. The early seventeenth century saw the emergence of an agnotology of flesh-based medicines; the early eighteenth century saw its fall.

MUMIA RETURNS

In the 1620s oath, theriac was mentioned in the same breath as mumia; the fate of these two medicaments in Russia parted ways somewhere in the middle of the seventeenth century. Both were rehabilitated, but in different ways, following different timelines, and to a different degree. Mumia was mentioned extremely infrequently in the late seventeenth century, and only in a limited set of documents; there is no visible trace of it outside of the Apothecary Chancery. It appears in official Russian medical documents in the 1730s, but was mentioned less frequently, and in fewer varieties, than its erstwhile companion theriac. Like theriac, the shift in views of mumia also took place during the social changes of the late seventeenth and early eighteenth centuries, and we can link this evolution to changing attitudes to human corpses in this period. There was a marked difference in the status of mumia in Russia in the 1730s as opposed to the 1620s, but if theriac's rehabilitation was dramatic, mumia's was rather quieter.

I have been able to identify only two seventeenth-century documents mentioning the use of mumia. The first is an undated mid-seventeenth-century stock list: that document, divided up into chapter by the kinds of ingredients, lists mumia as one of eleven items in the chapter on animal products [*sumpta animaliius*], alongside several kinds of animal blood, and also beeswax (a separate chapter, on animal parts [*animaliur partes*], lists another thirty-three animal products).[89] The second document is a 146-page list of medicaments and other supplies purchased in Hamburg in 1693–94; one item listed is "mumie."[90] Extant Apothecary Chancery prescriptions do not mention mumia, nor do any of the records relating to unofficial medical practices. There was some mention of mumia in late seventeenth-century Russia, but those mentions were few and far between, and entirely restricted to Apothecary Chancery documents.

We can again pick up the trail of mumia in the Medical Chancellery records from the 1730s. In 1737, it appeared in multiple documents. It was in stock in the Admiralty Hospital in St Petersburg in January, in the Moscow pharmacy in October, and St Petersburg in September.[91] It was also listed among the medicaments sent with the army to Smolensk.[92] Again in 1737, on 28 September, "mumia vera" was a part of a long list the Medical Chancellery was to make available to twenty-five army regiments via the field pharmacy at Smolensk, for the following year.[93] The same variant of mumia was in stock in November 1737.[94] It was again in stock in the St Petersburg Pharmacy in 1750.[95] These seven mentions are hardly a huge spike given the great variety of medicaments the Medical Chancellery, following the example of the Apothecary Chancery, kept in stock, but nevertheless represent a notable uptick in the presence of mumia in official Russian medicine by the 1730s.

These documents also tell us something of the kind of mumia being used in official Russian medicine. Two of these records specify that the substance in question was *Mumia Vera*. There were various kinds of mumia circulating Western Europe: in 1580s Frankfurt one could buy *Mumia Arabus, Mumia Arabus Vulgaris* or *Mumia Graecorum*.[96] *Mumia Vera* is a contraction of the phrase *Mumia vera Aegyptiaca*, true Egyptian mummy. This designation, in use in Western Europe from at least the 1580s, was used to indicate that the powder in question was supposed to have been created from ancient Egyptian mummified corpses, as opposed to the mummy powder created from more recent human remains from the Middle East or Europe or mummy powder not made from human corpses.[97] When official Russian medicine began to use mumia, it began to use that substance created from ancient North African human remains.

As so often when following the trail of mumia in early modern Russia, we are here chasing absences, and absences are tricky to interpret. Given the uneven but substantial loss of documents, and the fact that numerous documents are effectively unreadable, we cannot say definitively what the real level of mumia use was in late seventeenth- and early eighteenth-century Russia. We can, however, use the extant mentions of other substances to make comparisons. In 1737–40, we can identify six documents referencing mumia compared with ten that mention theriac, and more than thirty that mention one or more of the American plants guaiacum, jalap, sassafras, sarsaparilla, and Peruvian balsam.[98] At the least, we can say that mumia, at the height of its popularity in the early eighteenth century, was a less regular part of official Russian medicine than both theriac and American plant medicaments.

The growing yet still limited incorporation of mumia into official Russian medicine occurred at the same time as other changes to Russia's traditional ways of dealing with human remains. These changes were linked to major developments in the Russian Orthodox Church. In 1700, Patriarch Adrian, head of the Russian Orthodox Church, died, and instead of declaring a new patriarch, Peter the Great installed Stefan Iavorskii as an interim appointee.

This situation continued until the 1721 Spiritual Regulation, which created the Holy Synod, a governing committee of the Church that replaced the patriarch court, and so codified the submission of the church to the state. The church and state had never been entirely separate: the 1551 *Stoglav* Church council document was a collaboration between churchmen and the court; there was a department in the seventeenth-century chancery system dedicated to church affairs. Nevertheless, after 1721, the priorities of the Russian Orthodox Church were more closely aligned with those of the state than ever before.

This affected the treatment of corpses. Alongside official saints' cults approved of by the Russian Orthodox Church, before 1700 there had been several unofficial "corpse cults," local traditions involving the veneration of bodies not officially recognized as saints. According to Eve Levin, unofficial corpse cults had always had an uneasy relationship with the church hierarchy, and several were investigated in the sixteenth and seventeenth centuries. However, those early investigations tended towards verifying the holy status of the relics. The rearranged church under the Synod and the Spiritual Regulation increasingly cracked down on heterodox practices it saw as superstitious, including the unsanctioned saints' cults. This culminated in an investigation of 1744–45 and the suppression or attempted suppression of several such cults.[99] The period during which mumia was being brought into official Russian medicine was also the period in which the Russian state was attempting to re-regulate how human remains were treated.

A rather different development of early eighteenth-century Russia also affected Russians' views on mumia. In 1718, the Kunstkamera, a cabinet of curiosities collected by Peter the Great, opened its doors to the public in the new capital of St Petersburg. One of the most striking, if not shocking, parts of the Kunstkamera was the anatomical and zoological collection of the Dutchman Frederik Ruysch, purchased by Peter the Great during his earlier tour of Europe. This included the preserved remains of animals and humans, in particular those then considered "monstrous births," such as the skeletons of conjoined infants.[100] Not only were Russians to view anatomical specimens in the Kunstkamera, they were to help collect them: in 1718 Peter decreed that Russians were to provide such "monsters" to the Kunstkamera, and were encouraged to send in both living and dead specimens.[101] Through the Kunstkamera, Russians became familiar with the display of human remains, a stark contrast to the Russian Orthodox insistence of the previous century on swift and final burial.

The logic upon which Peter the Great's decree on monsters was made is important. Describing the "monsters" he wanted brought to the capital, he said the following:

> Ignorant [people] hide [them], believing that such monsters are born from the actions of the Devil, through witchcraft and curses. This is impossible, because the sole Creator of all creations is God and not the Devil, who has no power over such creations [as those monsters]. Rather, [those monsters occur] because of internal injuries, and also the fear and opinions of the mother during pregnancy, as there are many examples of how, when the mother is frightened, the marks [of that] can be found on the child.[102]

Peter the Great then saw contemporary Russian ideas about the role of the devil in creating "monsters" as superstition, the same logic the Synod would later use to condemn unofficial corpse cults. Peter here followed common early modern European thought on how the experiences of pregnant women, including such mundane acts as viewing paintings, could shape the fetus.[103] In the first half of the eighteenth century, there was pressure from Peter the Great and his officials to revise views on living and dead bodies away from ideas about good and evil towards what they believed was a more pragmatic understanding of cause and effect.

The success of Peter the Great's attempts to shift attitudes about human bodies can be seen through the key issues of autopsies and burials. Peter instituted autopsies, an expansion of the Apothecary Chancery policy of post-mortem examinations that had been so vigorously opposed less than a century earlier. He also introduced public dissections, another new way in which Russian society encountered dead bodies, and encouraged the embalming of bodies before burial, something very rarely practised in Russia before 1700.[104] Anthony Anemone has discussed what we can discern of Russian reactions to the Kunstkamera collections, anatomies, and embalming, emphasizing the varied responses. On the one hand, the Kunstkamera was hugely popular and full of visitors from the beginning, and some Russians did indeed send in specimens for the collection. On the other hand, members of the Imperial family refused to be embalmed and insisted on traditional Russian Orthodox Christian burial, and at least some of those who were required to attend Peter's autopsies were revulsed by the practice.[105] In the first half of the eighteenth century, Peter the Great pursued several policies that sought to force Russians to view human remains in practical, not moral, terms. The success of this was limited, but that limited success did cause some shift in how Russian society dealt with dead bodies.

As with theriac, the agnotology of flesh-based medicines that excluded mumia from medical use and knowledge in early modern Russia began to change as the Russian attitudes that had created that agnotology began to change. Key to these were shifts in how human remains were treated. Veneration of corpses was more closely regulated, autopsies used more extensively, and embalming introduced. St Petersburg society could experience those new practices by visiting the Kunstkamera or a public dissection. All of these changes were underpinned by an official drive to get rid of "superstition" and move ideas of the human body from a moral to a practical understanding. Mumia, which had been condemned a century before as ritually unclean, could then be rehabilitated as just another medicine the ingredients of which were neither evil nor good but merely useful.

CONCLUSION

Looking at medical drugs tells us about the recipients of drugs, in this case, Muscovite bodies. For early modern Russia, dominated by Russian Orthodox Christianity even as it was a multi-ethnic, multi-faith empire, the Muscovite body was the body created by God, and so had to be treated by God's rules. That meant a strict list of approved and disallowed consumables, some of which rules were arranged by ritual time, others of which were constant. It also meant treating dead human bodies correctly, keeping them intact and burying them swiftly and respectfully. Living and dying in a Christian body required constant maintenance and vigilance to stay in God's graces.

That maintenance significantly affected the prescriptions of medicaments. Both Russian and Western European documents show that certain medicines approved of in Western Europe were restricted in early modern Russia and restricted for religious reasons. Key among these were the global flesh-based medicines of theriac and mumia, both considered unclean by Muscovite officials, who banned the Western European medical practitioners of the Apothecary Chancery from using them. In the early seventeenth century, this was a significant restriction on medicine, and neither of these two vital parts of the Western European medical canon appear until the mid-seventeenth century. This can be seen as the kind of agnotology discussed by Schiebinger, a culturally induced rejection and ignorance of a kind of *materia medica.* In a fight between science and society, society won.

And then, society changed. At the same time as Blumentrost and Gurchin were beginning to grain traction promoting chemical medicine, Russian society of the very late seventeenth century began to metamorphose. Among the changes of that period was the emergence of a different attitude towards corpses in particular and human bodies more generally, which Peter the Great attempted to present as objects of scientific study, not religious beliefs. These changes, both medical and societal, made something of a space for theriac and, to a lesser extent, for mumia as well. Agnotologies, created by cultural values, can also be modified and even destroyed as cultural values themselves change. Within the Muscovite cosmology of Russian Orthodox Christianity, the materiality and status of the human body was key, and so materials of medicine always had to interact with rules about human bodies that came from society, not just science.

5

The New Textual Authorities

Thus far we have discussed materials like plants, chemicals, and bodies. There is one more vital group of objects for early modern medicine we must address: texts. Texts are, after all, objects. Tara Hamling and Catherine Richardson devoted an entire section of their edited volume on pre-modern material culture, *Everyday Objects*, to exactly this kind of material.[1] There is a whole branch of material culture studies devoted to the materialities of paper, paperwork, archives, manuscripts, scrolls, printed texts, and books of all kinds.[2] Paper or vellum is the raw material that is first created, then manipulated into the shape and format required, further changed by being written on by objects such as quills, and finally bound together with glue, thread, wax, and wooden or leather covers. These material processes of texts are culturally dependent: early modern texts were bound together in East Asia in a very different manner than that practised in Western Eurasia.[3] Muscovites owned, and made, texts according to their specific requirements. From Apothecary Chancery scrolls to the printed Western European texts in that department's library to hand-written Russian-language medical books, texts were the key materials, and are the only extant objects, of Muscovite medicine.

There were several different kinds of texts used in Muscovite medicine. Central to this study are the scrolls [pl. *stolptsy*, sing. *stolbets*], the Muscovite format for official documents, long, coarsely edged narrow strips of paper inscribed in black ink and glued end to end into a ticker-tape bureaucratic record.[4] The long strands were fundamental to this kind of textual material culture, as signatures on the back of each join served to verify the chain, and prevent documents being illicitly included or excluded. This practice tied together documents within the department, in Latin and in Russian, and departmental documents with those elsewhere in the bureaucracy, binding the empire together one dab of glue at a time. Alongside those scrolls were bound, Western-European-format manuscript books, beginning with the Slavonic *Garden of Health*, a format connected to the scrolls by the manner in which the text itself was produced but distinct in the wider format of the sewn-together gatherings of pages, the common use of headings in red, the occasional use of manuscript illustrations, and the hard bindings in wood and leather.[5] This form, originally coexisting with the scrolls, began to marginalize that latter information technology at the start of the eighteenth century, as official records were moved into this bound format. As this new kind of bureaucratic manuscript took hold, so did printed Russian-language medical books, produced by a modified version of the Western European movable type press, a technological shift that in turn increasingly marginalized the Slavic manuscript book. Yet manuscript medical books were used and even recopied well into the nineteenth century. Muscovite medical textual objects gradually Westernized in format along with the rest of elite Russian society, but manuscript practices were B movie vampires, endlessly returning from their supposed final resting place.

Considering texts as objects points us toward the processes of their creation, the form they took, and the role they played in the early modern Russian bureaucracy.[6] All the texts we have considered in this book were created collaboratively. They were the product of multiple hands – medical experts, translators, and scribes – and brought together summaries of information from other texts by other authors. They could be multilingual in origin, but the final version always privileged Russian. They were texts to be distributed, sometimes being part of a paperwork chain between different official departments, sometimes books to be read by medical experts or laypersons. And in the case of the Apothecary Chancery, such texts were commonly about *materia medica*. The creation and use of Muscovite texts bound together ideas, authors, objects, and audiences.

Here, we see another way in which the Apothecary Chancery was deeply involved in the globality of early modern medicine. The ideas in Apothecary Chancery texts were from broad traditions circulating throughout Afro-Eurasia, such as Eastern Church views on living and dead humans, the humoral composition of those same bodies, and the role of chemicals in healing them. Those documents cited widely, making specific references to recent medical authors like Paracelsus and van

Helmont, ancient world authorities like Hippocrates, Galen, and Plato, and discussing medical practices from India to Brazil. Botanicals from East and South Asia and the Americas, gums and coffee from West Africa, powdered mummies from Egypt, were contemplated and regulated in Slavic documents and wrapped up in a Muscovite paperwork package for the benefit of a Russian elite audience. In the Apothecary Chancery, paper objects defined the local limits of global medicine.

These processes were shaped by official views on literacy. Official clerks were required to be literate as it was a part of their job. Clergymen were generally expected to be literate, but non-literate clergy did exist.[7] The Russian nobility, whose traditional role was conducting warfare and advising the tsar via spoken counsel, only gradually adopted the cultural artifact of elite literacy from Western Europe during the early modern period. Although tsars and some nobles began to be interested in literacy from at least the 1670s, it took until the middle decades of the eighteenth century for literacy to be assumed as an automatic trait of a Russian noble. Outside of those groups, literacy was seen as suspicious. Valerie Kivelson has shown that possession of texts was a major reason individuals were caught up in witchcraft trials in the seventeenth century, as those with no official reason for owning books were suspected of using them for illicit purposes like malefic magic.[8] Those views began to change in the late seventeenth and early eighteenth centuries, but the connection between texts and officialdom remained strong. Even as we begin to see more texts aimed at a lay audience, those texts were often created by institutions or individuals linked to official circles. Texts are often called a kind of authority on ideas; in early modern Russia they were also an expression of and link to political authority.

The seventeenth century bequeathed those texts, and that textual tradition of how they were created and used, to the eighteenth century. The texts owned by the Apothecary Chancery were sent to the Academy of Sciences after that was founded in 1725; many are still to be found in that institution's library. The textual practices of the Apothecary Chancery, such as investigations where multiple departments collaborated via exchanging official reports, were also gifted to the eighteenth century. Looking at investigations and legislation on pharmacy from 1700 to 1750, we can find both direct links to earlier events and a clear continuation of Apothecary Chancery procedures we saw as early as 1628. Those traditions did change: there were new institutions, the new capital St Petersburg, and a new technology of text creation in printing. Yet the essence remained the same. The textual practices of eighteenth-century Russian official medicine were ultimately those of the seventeenth-century Apothecary Chancery.

AUTHORSHIP AND INTERTEXTUALITY

A major feature of reports, one of the kinds of texts upon which the Apothecary Chancery particularly relied, was intertextuality. Apothecary Chancery reports always answered a specific question but did so using reference to a broad range of knowledge, ideas, and texts. In doing so, these texts situated themselves in an explicit or hidden intertextual relationship with other texts created within or outside of the Russian Empire. That intertextuality was bound up with the complex authorship of the reports, as they were created through a process involving department heads, medical experts, translators, and scribes. Those reports cover a wide range of subjects, including the use of astrology in medicine, the virtues of venesection, the results of post mortems, the causes and symptoms of angina, how the actions of intestinal worms affect the human body, and the medicinal properties of deer horn.[9] We can examine the intertextuality and authorship of these varied documents through reports conventionally attributed to the British Apothecary Chancery employee Samuel Collins, but closer examination of which reveals a more complex process of composition.

The materiality of Collins's texts points us towards that complex authorship, and to how Collins's work was only part of a process, a part that was subsumed within Russian paperwork practices. Apothecary Chancery reports were created as scrolls, long strands of documents attached together. As we look at these strands, the Latin draft always sticks out. It is written on thinner paper than the Russian sections, and while the Russian sections are fairly regularly sized thin rectangles, the Latin sections are on paper of slightly different dimensions, up to one-third wider than the rest of the scroll.[10] To incorporate that Latin section into the rest of the scroll, Russian bureaucrats then manipulated it in three ways. First, the bottom of each sheet of the Latin text was glued to the start of the next page, whether that following page was in Latin or Russian. Second, the back of the join was signed by a Russian bureaucrat, a measure against illicit removals from or insertions into this official record. Thirdly, the oversized Latin page was folded to fit the dimensions of the Russian pages. Because of this last step, and the thinner paper of the Latin pages, text has been lost along the folds as holes have been worn in the document. Collins's contribution was physically transformed, and even partly destroyed, by the process of incorporating it into official Russian documentation practices.

Collins's reports were also changed in content during the production process. In 1665 he composed a report on valerian root, which covered the physical appearance, properties, methods of preparation, and modes of consumption of the plant.[11] As was the case with all reports, the Latin draft was translated into Chancery Russian for consumption by Russian bureaucrats, typically including the Apothecary Chancery director and often directors of other departments and sometimes even the tsar and his council. In this case, the final Russian version of the valerian root report substantially differs from the Latin draft: following the translation of Collins's text there is an additional section, introduced in the report as excerpts from a Russian herbal (described only as the herbal with 520 chapters) concerning the properties of valerian root. The final, Russian-language version of the report then provides more information than the Latin draft, adding practical knowledge in the form of a recipe from an herbal to the more general information that Collins provided.

Significant here is how the final, Russian-language version of the report came to differ from the Latin draft. Collins, who knew very little Russian, could not have chosen those excerpts to accompany his report. They then must have been chosen by a Russian-speaking member of the Apothecary Chancery staff, perhaps the scribe who prepared the final version of Collins's report. Given that we know there were multiple herbals owned by the Apothecary Chancery, it also seems likely that the (as yet unidentified) herbal was from the department's library. That herbal, described in the text as Russian-language, would then have been compiled by another Russian speaker, and most likely including information taken from earlier such texts. It is easy to ascribe the contents of the Apothecary Chancery reports to the physician whose name is always so prominently attached to them. Yet the valerian root document shows that we should instead see these documents as necessarily a collaborative product, a process in which the Russian members of the Apothecary Chancery played a substantial role in shaping the content of the text.

The Russian scribe who added the extra section to the report on valerian root was able to do so because the report summarized existing knowledge in other texts, and so it was appropriate for excerpts from other works to be added. This was also the case for other reports. One of those was coffee. Apparently only first being consumed as a drink of roasted beans in its original growing region, the Horn of Africa, sometime in the fifteenth century, coffee was known in the Ottoman Empire, Safavid Iran, and Europe by the late sixteenth century, but it was the seventeenth century that saw its precipitous rise in popularity, and the accompanying proliferation of coffee houses. The same century saw the creation of coffee plantations in Dutch-controlled Java, far from the original growing region. That burst of popularity for this beverage was fuelled by the production of works on the uses of coffee in multiple different languages.[12]

In 1664, Samuel Collins wrote a report on this fashionable drink. Collins's report begins with a geographical overview of coffee consumption. He states that it is in use by the Persians, Turks, and English, and that London now has 200 coffee houses.[13] He also notes the best methods of preparing coffee (with nutmeg and sugar), and the benefits of the drink including, of course, "многосоние отгоняет" – "[it] drives away much sleep." The origin of these assertions is unclear: unlike Collins's other reports, where he cites medical authorities such as Hippocrates, here no attribution is given.[14] It is perhaps significant that Collins had recently visited London, in 1662. As well as perhaps sampling some coffee at one of the coffee houses he mentioned, he may also have read about it. In 1662, the Royal Society, with which Collins had significant links, deposited "Discourses about Cyder and Coffee," in their archive, a text that certainly would have been of use to Collins when he wrote his report only two years later.[15] Collins here does not explicitly record the intertextual links of his report, but their existence can be inferred by the contents of his work.

As with the valerian root report, the final Russian version of the coffee text also differs from the Latin. Again, there is an addition, although much shorter than that inserted into the valerian root text. At the start of the text, the Russian version inserts the comment that "coffee is the berry of certain bushes that grow in Arabia," similar to how many Russian translations of this period inserted clarifications where the translators felt they were needed.[16] This is a little odd. Coffee is from the Horn of Africa, to the south of the Arabian Peninsula. We can shed light on this apparent mistake by looking at contemporary works on coffee. Nabil Matar has shown that British writers commonly referred to coffee as the "Arabian berry," in an attempt to demonize it through associations with Muslims in the anti-Islamic society of majority-Christian early modern Britain.[17]

Coffee was unfamiliar to Russians at this time: this is the first known mention of it in a Russian text; a limited number of coffee houses would appear in Russia only half a century later, in the 1720s, and the beverage was not really popular there until the twentieth century.[18] It then seems improbable that Russian scribes would be able to make such an addition themselves. On the other hand, Collins would have been aware of how other British people referred to coffee. The addition was added in Russian, so it is likely to have occurred as the result of a conversation between the translator and Collins. The hidden intertextuality of Apothecary Chancery reports was then partly created by the oral context in which textual production took place.

Although much of the intertextuality of the Apothecary Chancery reports was hidden and unacknowledged, there were some explicit citations. In 1665, Samuel Collins co-created yet another report, this time on obesity.[19] This is typically interpreted as a pointed comment directed toward Tsar Aleksei Mikhailovich, who, despite his careful adherence to Muscovite fasting traditions, was apparently somewhat corpulent. In his report, Collins explicitly cites Hippocrates's views on obesity – he frames certain of his points about the health risks of obesity as "according to Hippocrates' understanding" [*po Ippokratovu razumeniiu*] – linking his own opinions to this great medical authority of the ancient world. According to Michael Stolberg, this was typical of early modern European authors tackling this subject: he attributes the distinct similarities of early modern works on the topic of obesity to their close adherence to Hippocrates's views on the subject.[20] We can then see that reports which were drafted by Samuel Collins relied on several other groups of texts: Russian-language herbals, British works on coffee, and ancient world medical texts.

Apothecary Chancery reports were complex creations. Each answered a specific, discrete question, but in order to do so relied upon multiple texts and individuals. The medical practitioner or practitioners involved, like Samuel Collins, would consult works on the subject that would then feed into the draft Latin report either explicitly or in hidden ways. A translator would then create the final, Russian version, sometimes in conversation with the creator of the draft to tweak its content in the process. Finally, a scribe or translator could sometimes add further content by reference to other, Russian-language, texts on the same subject. Reports, so important to the functioning of the Apothecary Chancery and its role in the Russian imperial bureaucracy, were co-constructed by multiple authors with access to multiple texts.

AUTHENTICATING UNICORN HORN

The intertextuality of Apothecary Chancery reports affected how other, non-paper, materials were treated. Despite the department's notable dislike of certain flesh-based medicines like theriac and mummia, one non-fleshy animal product was the focus of considerable interest at the Russian court. That object was unicorn horn. Across the seventeenth century, the court acquired multiple objects then believed to be the horns of land unicorns for both decorative and medicinal purposes. Those objects were hugely expensive, and so it fell to Apothecary Chancery experts to authenticate specific examples of unicorn horn via experiments taken from early modern Western Europe's extensive literature on the subject. This was unique. No extant Apothecary Chancery document mentions any other experiments on, or tests of, materials held by the department. In order to understand how and why texts were linked to experiments on objects, we need to look at the history of this object called unicorn horn within and outside of the Apothecary Chancery.

Multiple Apothecary Chancery documents mention unicorn horn [*rog edinoroga*]. Powdered unicorn horn was a trusted enough ingredient to be prescribed to the tsar himself in 1645.[21] It was then prescribed several more times in the 1650s–1660s, always to members of court, making it a high-status medicine.[22] Unicorn horn also appears in multiple trade documents from this period: four times in the 1650s–1680s the Russian court purchased, or were offered the opportunity to purchase, one or more horns.[23] According to foreign sources, there were also other instances when the Russian court was offered unicorn horn for purchase: in the 1610s the Italian merchant Pietro della Valle offered the Russians a horn found on Greenland.[24] In contrast to the concern over, and restrictions on, the fleshy medical drugs in the early to mid-seventeenth century, Russians were very happy to buy and consume unicorn horn.

As early modern Christians, Russians believed in the existence of unicorns as a part of their belief in the Bible as literally true. When the Bible was translated into Greek the Hebrew word רְאֵם [*re'em*] was rendered as *monoceros*, and from there later into the Latin equivalent term, *unicornis* in medieval European Christian editions.[25] Consequently, the word "unicorn" appears in early modern editions such as the King James – and the East Slavic – Bible no less than seven times; modern English translations of the Bible instead translate this word as "wild ox."[26] As the unicorn was mentioned in the Bible, so the belief of the time ran, then it must have existed in the biblical period.[27] Moreover, contemporary thinking went, as nothing created by God can ever be fully destroyed, unicorns must still exist. To the early modern Christian, the Bible's standing on the unicorn represented absolute authority: the Bible mentions the unicorn, therefore the unicorn must exist. Even Ambroise Paré, influential French surgeon and arch-critic of superstition and nonsense everywhere, who had significant doubts about the unicorn and the medicinal properties of its horn, nevertheless stated that it must exist, as the Bible says that it does.[28] It was only over the course of the eighteenth century that the existence of the unicorn was generally considered to have been disproven, and objects that had previously been labelled as unicorn horn reclassified as originating from other creatures.[29] To most modern people, unicorns are a myth; to early modern Christians, they were real flesh and blood creatures.

Early modern Christians also found support for the existence of unicorns in other texts. The Roman naturalists Pliny the Elder and Claudius Aelianus discussed the unicorn, as did the Greek physician Ctesias of Cnidus. However, there were issues in the ancient world discussions of the unicorn. Pliny the Elder, Claudius Aelinus, and Ctesias of Cnidus all describe the unicorn differently, including giving contradictory accounts of what the horn should look like. Even more importantly, other ancient world authorities were disinterested in the topic: Aristotle devoted little attention to the subject, and Galen ignored it entirely.[30] Ancient world authors do differ on various subjects, and not all authors interested in medicine and natural history cover all the same subjects. Yet for major authors like Aristotle and Galen to ignore the issue, and others to hold wildly varying views on the basic appearance of a creature, is still somewhat unusual. Early modern readers were confident that unicorns existed, yet authoritative ancient world texts were not clear on what, exactly, a unicorn was.

Not only were notes on unicorns included in the Bible and ancient world natural historical texts, material traces of unicorns could be found as well. Across the medieval and early modern period, "unicorn horns" were bought and sold. The value and function of unicorn horns were bound up with the complicated history of what they were and what they signified. This powerful and single-horned beast became a symbol of Christ, and so was thought to have similar properties of purity inherent to the body and the blood of Christ, objects consumed by Catholics during mass. Unicorn horns became prized as protecting from poison, curing any disease, and also as ornaments for royalty. Of those still in existence, we can see that many such horns were the narwhal's distinctive long, white tusk with spiral markings; some other supposed land unicorn horns were from rhinoceroses. The narwhal tusks were sold in particular by the Danes, who made such a profit in this trade that they created a throne from the tusks to show off the source of their wealth. Here, the Danes were being knowingly dishonest about the kind of unicorn they were selling. The narwhal was then understood as a "sea unicorn"; the Danes sold those tusks as the horns of the "land unicorn." And, due to the substantial prices these horns fetched, others were faked, with different kinds of horns manipulated to create the spiral markings that increasingly came to be seen as the true mark of the unicorn.[31] When the Apothecary Chancery was buying unicorn horns, it was engaging in a widespread, but problematic, trade.

As in other instances when the Apothecary Chancery was concerned about medical drugs, in the case of the precious but often-faked unicorn horns reports were composed to discuss the issue. Reports on alicorns – another name for unicorn horns – were produced in 1655, 1657, 1658, and 1669.[32] This period is particularly rich in extant Apothecary Chancery reports: during the same period the department produced the reports on coffee and valerian root, as well as texts on various animal parts and their possible uses in medicines.[33] Yet the Apothecary Chancery medical practitioners were also following a pan-European trend regarding writing about unicorns in the mid-seventeenth century. Odell Shepard, in his noteworthy study of the unicorn in Europe, states that at least twenty-five entire books or chapters in natural-philosophical tracts were dedicated to the land unicorn during the sixteenth and seventeenth centuries.[34] When the Apothecary Chancery wrote about unicorn horn, it was engaging with an established topic within natural historical literature.

Indeed, the Apothecary Chancery texts explicitly rely on earlier sources, in particular early modern Western European texts: Alexander Lichifinus's 1657 Apothecary Chancery report describes the unicorn on the basis of statements by Marco Polo, and also Andrea Bacci, a sixteenth-century papal physician.[35] Andreas Engelhardt, writing an accompanying report in the same year, similarly relied upon the substantial Western European tradition of thought on unicorns.[36] Despite dealing with a known substance – the department was sure enough about unicorn horn to have prescribed it to the tsar more than a decade earlier – these 1657 reports are substantial: they cover where unicorns are to be found, what true unicorn horn looks like, its medicinal uses, and, crucially, which experiments have been developed to establish the veracity and potency of any particular horn. Here, then, is the crux of the mid-seventeenth-century unicorn horn reports: they were designed to help the department buy authentic, efficacious horn.

The driving forces behind these reports were Russian bureaucrats. We know this as it was standard department practice for the department head to order reports on a specific topic; we can also see this in the distinct reluctance and skepticism expressed by the foreign medical practitioners like Lichifinus and Engelhardt as they phrased their reports. Engelhardt wrote: "[c]oncerning the monoceros, or unicorn, ancient philosophers have dreamed up varied and surprising things, and such [creations] are highly repugnant to current scholarship."[37] Both authors even went as far as noting their opposition to writing on such a subject, with Lichifinus writing "[m]any doctors informed us [of things concerning the unicorn], in which it is impossible to believe, but, in short, he, the doctor, will complete his business," and Engelhardt stating that "about such [matters] he, the doctor, finds it inappropriate to write, were it not for the fact that it is about such [a matter] that he has been commanded to write, and he does so [only] in connection to this [command]."[38] Engelhardt and Lichifinus were the men whose names are listed on the reports as authors, but the content of those texts was taken from earlier works, and the very existence of the Apothecary Chancery documents on this subject is due to Russian bureaucrats, not the foreign physicians.

This reluctantly given advice on how to verify your unicorn horn was put into practice. In an unprecedented and never-repeated action, on 25 June 1658 the Apothecary Chancery carried out an experiment to test the horn they were considering purchasing. Two of the men who had written reports on the unicorn – Doctors Lichifinus and Engelhardt – alongside two apothecaries – Christian Eichler and Robert Benyon – carried out the following experiment. The test was conducted on three doves: the first dove was given arsenic; the second was given arsenic and then (powdered) unicorn horn; the third was given the horn and then arsenic. The first time around, all the doves survived. The experiment was then repeated, and the first and second doves died, and the third survived.[39] The second experiment was judged to be a success, and the horn was declared to be genuine and efficacious.

The dove experiment – one of the "poison trials," as Alisha Rankin calls them – carried out by the Apothecary Chancery was also described and performed elsewhere in Europe.[40] The Italian doctor Girolamo Cardano wrote about it in 1559, nearly a century before the Apothecary Chancery performed it, and Odell Shepard considers that thereafter this experiment became the most popular method by which to test the horn. Certainly, it was carried out several times across early modern Europe in the century or so after Cardano's text was published: in 1573 Andrea Bacci wrote that the Cardinal of Trent carried out that experiment in Italy; Ambroise Paré wrote about carrying out this and other experiments regarding the horn in France in his 1582 tract "Discourse on the Unicorn" (but expressed his dissatisfaction with all such experiments); in 1636 the apothecary John Woldenburg carried out the experiment in Copenhagen, Denmark, before an audience including the noted natural historian Ole Worm.[41] Looking at unicorn horn in the Apothecary Chancery shows us how texts linked intellectual communities together in their treatments of materials. This shared tradition of writings on the land unicorn and its horn led these various figures across early modern Europe to use the identical processes to come to often similar conclusions regarding the properties of related objects.

Tests of unicorn horn and texts on unicorn horn tell us about the Apothecary Chancery's use of documents to understand and control materials. On one occasion, the Apothecary Chancery used documents they created, based on texts other people had created, to carry out an experiment to determine the quality of a natural object. On multiple other occasions, the Apothecary Chancery used only their texts, based on earlier works on the same subject, to understand their *materia medica*. Texts were a part of physically engaging with a material, recommending its use or practices for verifying it; they were always key to understanding and controlling those objects. In the seventeenth century, this control was primarily exercised within the department, but by the early eighteenth century this control began to edge into the Moscow medical market.

LEGISLATING THE MARKET

Throughout the seventeenth century, the Apothecary Chancery used texts to record and create official knowledge on global medicinal objects; by the early eighteenth century those paperwork practices would also be used to legislate the use of medicinal objects outside of the department. As we saw in chapter 1, particularly in the second half of the century they were increasingly involved in investigating both medical malpractice and malefic magic. Notably, the role of the Apothecary Chancery in those trials was to examine objects, consult texts, and produce reports, which reports in turn informed the creation of other official texts. The large-scale investigations of the Kitai-gorod markets in the 1690s led to legislative action in the early eighteenth century. There had been earlier legislation regarding the private sale of medicines: Aleksei Mikhailovich had restricted some such sales in 1673; the 1685 Apothecary Chancery investigation refers to a system of approving certain medicaments for sale.[42] Nevertheless, the legislative actions taken by Peter the Great in the 1700s were significant, as they were by far the most extensive pharmacy legislation to date, and legislation that directly drew on the Apothecary Chancery's work. That action took the shape of hand-written decrees regarding the sale of medical drugs and licences for private pharmacists that laid out rules for Moscow's medical marketplace, continuing the prioritization of manuscripts we see in the seventeenth-century chancery system.[43] The paperwork practices of the seventeenth-century Apothecary Chancery directly fed into the legislative texts of the early eighteenth century.

We can trace the Apothecary Chancery's involvement in trials back to the 1628 Loptunov witchcraft trial we looked at in chapter 1.[44] That case provided a model for the department's future involvement in such cases: another part of the chancery system arrested someone with suspicious natural objects, those objects were sent for the Apothecary Chancery experts to examine, based on that examination and the consultation of texts in their library the department then produced an official, written report on the item, which was then used as expert testimony during the legal procedure. Following that 1628 case, the department was then involved in five more witchcraft cases between the 1650s and the 1700s.[45] Across the same time period, they also used the same practices of consulting texts and producing written reports to participate in the prosecution of medical malpractice, including the final big case of the century which began in 1685 and continued on into the 1690s that took a broad look at the unofficial medicines on sale on the Kitai-gorod markets.[46] The reports of the Apothecary Chancery regarding this final investigation formed the basis of early eighteenth-century Petrine pharmacy legislation.

In November 1701 Peter the Great announced the establishment of eight new private apothecary shops to be located in some of the busiest areas of Moscow, including one near the herb markets of Kitai-gorod, the capital's major trading district and epicentre of the malpractice cases over private medical sales of the previous few decades.[47] The aim of these new apothecary shops was explicitly laid out in Peter's order, which states:

> In the imperial city of Moscow henceforth [there will be] other, new, apothecary shops, so that the herb market, that [is] in Kitai-gorod, and also stalls on every street and crossroads, from which inappropriate herbs and simples[48] are sold instead of medicines, will no longer exist, and they will be destroyed and cleared away from all streets and crossroads, and in those herb markets, other wares will be traded, in which it is appropriate to trade.[49]

The "inappropriate herbs and simples" Peter mentions are a reference to the physical evidence examined as a part of the 1690s medical malpractice cases involving the Kitai-gorod market. This decree, and the licences of the eight new apothecaries that would follow, were an attempt to control private pharmacy practices through official texts informed by Apothecary Chancery reports.

Echoing Peter's order of 1701, the licence given to the new apothecaries reiterates the role of the new, licensed, pharmacies in pushing out the herb markets and establishing a new kind of medicine:

> In that, that is to say, his [the licensed pharmacist's] apothecary shop, all medicines made by his workers in his presence will make a great loss for the criminal Vegetable and Apothecary and Herb Markets, and in accordance with the order of the father of our Great Sovereign Aleksei Mikhailovich on the 28th February 1673,[50] apothecary medicines created in the Apothecary Chancery which are sold in the Old and in the New Pharmacies,[51] [such as] internal elixirs, vodkas and oils, those aforementioned market stalls are forbidden to stock

> and to sell, and whosoever [of the market traders] dares to stock and to sell [such medicines], they will be harshly punished.[52]

The licence goes on directly to blame the sale of medicines by these herb markets for the recent deaths, such as of Prince Fedor Shcherbatskii in 1679 and boyar P.P. Saltykov in 1699.[53]

> And now in those markets traders stock and sell such pharmaceutical medicines, [which are] falsely created, and all types of oils, and from their sale of medicines abnormalities and harm and untimely loss is caused [which affects] many people . . . [thus] it is forbidden to trade in apothecary medicines and oils in such aforementioned markets, so that all people will be protected from harm and from the untimely loss caused by such unskilled practices.[54]

The establishment of the new private apothecary shops was thus explicitly framed in terms of previous abuses by stallholders in selling inappropriate medicines, specifically the kinds of internal and compound medicines that previously were only legally created in the Apothecary Chancery. The new apothecary shops, then, were established in order to supply the ordinary denizens of Moscow with safe internal and compound drugs.

It took twelve years following the 1701 decree to open all planned eight new apothecary shops in Moscow; it would only be in 1721 that Peter the Great authorized the opening of similar shops in St Petersburg and other Russian cities.[55] In Moscow, the process was overseen by the Apothecary Chancery, which was tasked with examining and licensing the pharmacists. Indeed, the first two licences (granted in 1701) were both to employees of the Apothecary Chancery, Johann Gotfried (Gregorius) and Daniel Gurchin.[56] Gregorius's shop was to be located in the new Foreign Suburb, and Gurchin's in Belgorod, not far from Kitaigorod, the centre of the problematic herbal medicines trade.[57] Johann Gotfried (employed in the department 1685/6–1700s), also known as Gregorius, was part of a dynasty of apothecaries who worked for the Apothecary Chancery. The department initially took him on as an apothecary student, paid for his studies abroad, and then hired him.[58] Gurchin's lineage of Russian service was not as long as Gotfried's, but evidence such as the medical texts he composed for the tsar and tsarevich along with a poem he composed on Peter's military victories demonstrate that he was committed to the glorification of his Russian masters.[59] In licensing Gotfried and Gurchin as the first private apothecaries, the Apothecary Chancery continued its policy of mobilizing its paperwork practices to intrude into Moscow's medical marketplace, and drawing upon loyal employees to do so.

The written reports of the seventeenth-century Apothecary Chancery fed directly into the creation of written legislation that led to the first licensed apothecaries in Moscow, both a continuation of Apothecary Chancery practice and the start of its undoing. The legislation itself, and the licences that followed, both explicitly cite the earlier cases investigated with the help of the Apothecary Chancery. The department then also examined and licensed the new pharmacists and provided two of its own employees as the first wave of newly licensed practitioners. The point of these changes was control of the medical marketplace by the government. As Apothecary Chancery texts had been used as a vital part of investigating the cases leading up to this change, texts influenced by the Apothecary Chancery's work were also the way in which the change was laid out. The textual practices of the Apothecary Chancery, previously used to understand materials and track investigations, were now also being used to control the medical marketplace.

THE LETTERS OF THE LAW

The view of private medical practice in early eighteenth-century Moscow in the 1701 legislation is fairly straightforward: the problematic medical markets have been removed and well-created drugs can be sourced from the licensed apothecaries. Move along please, there is nothing to see here. Yet further examination reveals a different picture, and one that allows us to see how the Apothecary Chancery's paperwork practices continued to exert an influence on Russian medicine long after the department was shuttered and the scrolls packed away.

Despite the 1701 legislation, there continued to be issues with private medical practitioners who created inappropriate or dangerous medical drugs well into the eighteenth century. Eighteenth-century Russian legislation created to deal with that ongoing problem shows a major shift in the materiality of legal documents. The legislation and licences from 1701 were all handwritten, as – with the sole exception of the 1649

Ulozhenie [Law Code] – were all official documents before 1714; decrees regulating medical and pharmacy practices from 1721, 1729, 1750, and after were all printed. Yet these printed laws did not signal the end of the manuscript tradition, or the end of the influence of the Apothecary Chancery. Rather, they were created with the manuscript practices inherited from the Apothecary Chancery and the Muscovite chancery system. Considering this history of medico-legal documents shows how manuscript shaped print.

The history of print in the East Slavic lands follows a different trajectory from that of print in East Asia or Western Europe. In the middle of the sixteenth century, two printers, Ivan Fedorov and Peter Mstislavets, were the experts behind a short-lived experiment that adapted the Western European press to Muscovite specifications. Often specifically attributed to the Moscow court, there was in fact a small circle of powerful elite figures who patronized their printing, leading to the creation of a number of Slavonic printed religious texts. The quality of the produced texts was not what Fedorov and Mstislavets's patrons wanted and so the project quietly ended, and printing fell out of fashion in the Russian Empire until the early eighteenth century.[60] Central to Fedorov and Mstislavets's efforts was how to make Cyrillic printable. They retained the Old Church Slavonic alphabet – a version of the Cyrillic alphabet that contains several letters not used in modern Russian – and carefully mimicked the contemporary script. In effect, they adapted the technology to the language.

After Fedorov and Mstislavets's ill-fated efforts, the conclusive introduction of print to Russia came, unsurprisingly, during the reign of that noted Westernizer, Peter the Great. In 1714, he ruled that all laws, passports, and other vital documents like blank forms were henceforth to be printed. As Simon Franklin has argued, Peter the Great used the fact that the state then owned the only press to reimagine this tool of mass publishing as a machine of social control, creating hard-to-fake official documents.[61] Rather than print religion, Peter printed law. Peter's approach differed from that of Fedorov and Mstislavets's project in one other notable way. In 1708, he had reformed the Russian language by introducing the *grazhdanka*, the civil script, which removed certain letters from the alphabet deemed extraneous.[62] This facilitated the printing introduced six years later, as it was easier to produce movable type in the reduced number of letters of this new Cyrillic alphabet. Fedorov and Mstislavets tried to adapt the press to the language; Peter adapted the language to the press. The pharmacy legislation of the 1720s and later was produced in exactly this revised and printable Russian language.

In 1721, the Senate in St Petersburg approved just such a new, printed law, in this case putting the Medical Chancellery in charge of newly established town apothecaries, requiring that department to help with the supply of medicaments to the provinces, and putting all hospitals under their purview.[63] At first glance, this decree looks like a new piece of Petrine legislation. It was put in place by the Senate (established in 1711) which met in St Petersburg, the new capital (founded in 1703), and entrusted affairs to the newly established Medical Chancellery. Indeed, a key part of this law was finally to hand over all remaining affairs of the Muscovite Apothecary Chancery to the Petrine Medical Chancellery. Yet behind this facade of novelties lies a deeper structure of substantial continuity with the Apothecary Chancery's earlier activities. As we saw above, the issue of regulating apothecaries was entrusted to the Apothecary Chancery only twenty years earlier. Indeed, the 1721 decree states that this is an expansion of the current system of licensed apothecaries that already exists for Moscow to St Petersburg and other cities of the empire, an implicit reference to the 1701 legislation and licences. That 1701 legislation was created on the basis of Apothecary Chancery investigations stretching back at least to the 1670s. Although the decree mentions other issues, such as the hospitals, it devotes significant space to the sourcing and provision of appropriate medicines, such a central part of the Apothecary Chancery's work. Also significantly, the Archiator of the Medical Chancellery who was instrumental in creating the 1721 law was Laurentius Blumentrost junior, son of Laurentius Blumentrost senior, key figure in the Apothecary Chancery. Despite the initial appearances, the Apothecary Chancery was still shaping the priorities, legislation, and personnel of official Russian medicine in 1721.

That 1721 decree takes up a page in the vital document collection *Complete Collection of Laws of the Russian Empire*; a later decree of 1729 takes up ten lines.[64] Despite its brevity, that 1729 law is also significant to understanding the legacy of the Apothecary Chancery. The decree states that those without proof of medical expertise [*ne imeiushchim svidetel'stv v znanii Meditsiny*] should not be allowed to practise medicine under threat of severe fines and punishments, and entrusts the enforcement of such to the Medical Chancellery, which is instructed to enforce these rules firmly [*nakrepko*].[65] This issue of proof of medical expertise again takes us back to the Apothecary Chancery: not only had the department been issuing licences to apothecaries from 1701, it had been examining potential staff members regarding their expertise since 1599.[66] A brief note from the late 1720s relating to the Medical Chancellery again shows an ongoing concern with the issues first dealt with by the Apothecary Chancery decades earlier.

Yet the clearest example of the ongoing influence of the Apothecary Chancery on official Russian medicine and printed decrees regarding medicine comes from 1748–50. The 1740s brought unexpected challenges to the legislative regime originally set up in 1701. The unlawful sale of medicines on the Kitai-gorod markets in Moscow once again caused problems and was linked to deaths. One case in particular caused a great stir, leading to a printed law re-regulating medical practice not merely in Moscow and St Petersburg, but in the entire Russian Empire.[67]

To understand the problem, we need to turn to the details of this case. The investigation surrounded the death of a police captain's wife in Moscow in 1748 after she had taken a medical drug sold to her by one Fedor Priadunov. Priadunov, a Schismatic [*raskol'nik*] Arkhangelsk merchant, was also implicated in the serious illnesses or deaths of several other patients. Whether or not he ever practised medicine in Arkhangelsk is unknown, and all the patients the investigation lists were residents of Moscow. After his arrest, samples of Priadunov's medicine were sent both to the main pharmacy in Moscow and to the Mining College in St Petersburg. The case as a whole was heard by the Senate, also in St Petersburg, with input from the Medical Chancellery, again also located in St Petersburg. The Senate finally decided against Priadunov, condemning him, and ordering the printing of a new law on the regulation of medical drugs in the entire empire.

Much of the Priadunov affair was new. Indeed, one aspect of the Priadunov case was unprecedented either in the seventeenth or the eighteenth century: unique of all the imperial Russian pharmacy legislation, the 1750 law not only describes the abuses it aimed to stop, but named and shamed the individual held responsible, Fedor Priadunov. This was unexpected. The names of the transgressive market sellers whose malpractice in the late 1690s led to the 1701 law banning the Kitai-gorod trade and establishing the new system of licensed apothecary shops were also known, and the 1701 law – and the resulting apothecary licences – goes into substantial detail about those transgressions. The markets themselves are mentioned as the site of the malpractice, yet no individual is named and shamed as Priadunov would be, half a century later. The Priadunov case was then in some ways a singular affair.

This odd case was heavily embedded in the new, eighteenth-century structures of the empire. The major institutions involved in the deliberation of his case – the Senate, the Medical Chancellery, the Mining College – were all eighteenth-century creations. Indeed, despite the fact that Priadunov had committed his alleged crimes in Moscow, several of the institutions that judged him were located in the new capital of St Petersburg. When the Senate had made its decision and written the new law, that decree was printed, following the practice established in 1714. The decree was created in 1750, and distributed across the Russian Empire, with copies going to the governor [*gubernator*] of each region – another Petrine innovation, established in 1708 to replace the *voevoda* system of military governors like the *voevoda* Fedor Matveevich Apraksin to whom Afanasii of Kholmogory had dedicated the *Extract from Doctors' Knowledge* some fifty years prior – along with instructions that it be publicly proclaimed and strictly enforced.[68] The method of producing the decree that condemned Priadunov, and the institutions that condemned him and promulgated and upheld the new law, were all eighteenth-century creations.

Yet other aspects of the Priadunov case reveal older trends. During this investigation, the Moscow pharmacy was ordered to put the medicine "to every test known to apothecary art" [*vo vsem ponadlezhashchemu aptekarskomu isskustvu osvedetelstvovat'*] to determine its composition.[69] This followed the precedent of the 1628 witchcraft trial, where botanical knowledge was used to determine that a root was medicinal; the 1657 unicorn horn experiment, conducted on the basis of authoritative texts on the subject; and the 1685 *pianoe zel'ia* case, which also revolved around the statements of trained medical experts who referred to canonical reference texts to examine a questionable medicament. Moreover, the 1750 decree explicitly cites both the 1721 and 1729 decrees, particularly on the point of banning those without evidence of medical knowledge from practising medicine; the decrees of the 1720s were themselves part of a legal tradition regulating pharmacy stretching back to the 1670s. The condemnation of Priadunov in 1750 was a part of the fraught history, going back decades, of the interactions of official and unofficial Russian medicine regulated by official examinations of the medicaments in question.

Most significantly, the Priadunov case file we find today in the Senate papers shows us the interaction of the manuscript and print traditions in official Russian medicine. Only the final page of the file is a printed document; the rest of the file is handwritten.[70] These manuscripts are not identical to Apothecary Chancery documents. Gone are the long, thin scrolls, replaced by Western European style folio sheets, copies of the documents sent back and forth between the different departments compiled into one official Senate record, pages divided into two columns and all bound into huge volumes that not even Tolstoy could outdo. The hand, too, is different: a smaller, blockier, and neater version of *skoropis* in comparison with the Apothecary Chancery's florid, sprawling script. Here, print did not replace manuscript. Rather, a single printed sheet emerged out of a multitude of manuscript pages. In the issue of Russian laws on medicine and pharmacy, print was the concise end product of an extensive process conducted in manuscript.

Following the letters of the law from 1701 to 1750 shows us the extent to which eighteenth-century official medicine depended upon earlier developments. The decrees of 1721 and after look different, as they were produced by a different information technology and relate to new institutions. Yet there is more continuity than is initially apparent. The 1750 decree is explicit in its relationship to the earlier decrees of 1721 and 1729, and the law of 1721 implicitly references the decree and licences of 1701, which in turn lead us back to the late seventeenth-century investigations that led to the creation of those documents. Moreover, the investigation that led to the 1750 decree used the same paperwork practice of collecting expert opinions from multiple branches of government in manuscript that the chancery system had used since at least 1628. The printed legislation of eighteenth-century Russia was not divided from the manuscript paperwork practices of the Apothecary Chancery; it emerged from it.

PRINTING ADVICE

As Russia was shifting the letters of the laws regarding medicine from manuscript to print, there was a similar development regarding medical texts for laypersons. In contrast to Western Europe, where the mass printing of texts emerged as the first stages of the print revolution, it was only after laws were printed in Russia that other texts, including self-help medical books, began to be printed. In the historiography of Russian medicine, there is a gaping chasm between manuscript and print: those of us who work on manuscripts typically work exclusively on handwritten documents, and almost all of us focus on the period before 1700; those who work on printed books similarly rarely use manuscripts, and largely concentrate on the second half of the eighteenth century.[71] Yet history is not so neat. The rise of printed popular works on medicine in Russia is entangled with the history of Russian medicine in manuscript, and, for historians is now further interwoven with later information technologies, as we increasingly access those manuscripts and printed texts via microfilms, scans, websites, JPEGs, and PDFs. Here we can turn to the physical and digital remains of early eighteenth-century popular Russian medical works to see how, instead of a chasm between the manuscript and print material worlds, there was a messy, contradictory, and incomplete shift from one information technology to another across the course of several decades.

The first two decades of the eighteenth century saw the continuation of the manuscript history of lay medical texts. Soon after his shop was established in 1701, Gurchin again began producing medical books. One such text was the *Pharmacy for Transport or Service,* composed in 1708 but extant in copies at least into the 1720s.[72] Gurchin was here using an information technology associated with the creation of a limited number of copies, but did so in a way that explicitly sought a wide audience for his works, his apothecary shop, and himself. The 1708 text begins:

> Pharmacy for Transport or Service. Compiled in a concise fashion from various apothecary or surgical books, for the good of service persons, and their horses, with which in the absence of a surgeon [they] might help themselves during any of their own or their horse's infirmities. Produced with the zeal and toil of His Highness the Tsar's apothecary Daniel Gurchin of the imperial city of Moscow in the year of our Lord 1708.[73]

According to S.M. Grombakh, a printed edition of this text was prepared but never produced.[74] This is entirely plausible, as other books were being printed in Russia in this period. One early Russian printed work – the *Alkoran o Magomete,* the first official (perhaps the first ever) Russian translation of the Quran – appeared in 1716, only two years after Peter the Great's decision to print decrees, and less than a decade after Gurchin's original version of the *Pharmacy for Transport or Service* appeared.[75] As the first Petrine printed books were being produced, Apothecary Chancery staff balanced on the edge of the two contemporary information technologies, creating medical books that circulated in manuscript and were planned to appear in print.

Soon after, medical books did indeed begin to be printed in Russia. Grombakh considers the first such work to be a 1719 work on the properties of medicinal waters.[76] It would take a little longer for works on medical drugs to appear in print. In 1738, the Academy of Sciences published the first Russian-language edition of Franz Philipp Florinus's 1702 German-language household guide *Oeconomus prudens et legalis*, as *Florin's Economy* [*Florinova Ekonomiia*].[77] Significantly for our purposes, this text includes several medical recipes. In this, the Academy of Sciences was following the Apothecary Chancery: not only did the Academy of Sciences inherit Apothecary Chancery's textual tradition when they were given the department's library, they also took on its role as a translator and creator of medical texts, including those for laypersons. Thirty years after Gurchin produced his *Pharmacy for Transport or Service* in manuscript, official departments were beginning to produce some Russian-language medical books in print.

The printing of medical books that began with those works of 1719 and 1738 would not truly take off into a broader endeavour until after 1760, and manuscript production of medical texts was far from immediately killed off by the first printed medical texts in Russia.[78] We have already looked at the manuscript book *Little Ark of Medicine*, produced in or after 1730.[79] There were also several self-help medical texts copied in manuscript across the eighteenth and even into the nineteenth century.[80] Some such works again take us back to the paperwork practices of the Apothecary Chancery. The Apothecary Chancery *Pharmacopoeia*, first compiled in 1676 and used and copied into the 1700s as an official medical text, was transformed into a lay medical guide in the early eighteenth century. The *Pharmacopoeia for Domestic Use*, as it is referred to, explicitly sets out its new purpose in its introduction, stating that it laid out medical recipes in such a way that "any person [will be able] to use [those medicines] for themselves in the absence of a doctor."[81] These domestic versions of the Apothecary Chancery *Pharmacopoeia* were copied into the nineteenth century.[82] Even as the printing presses of eighteenth-century Russia began to produce printed medical books, the established manuscript tradition continued to produce copies of existing texts and even created new works from old texts.

The *Pharmacopoeia, Pharmacy for Transport or Service, Little Ark of Medicine,* and *Florin's Economy* differ in their original materiality in that the first three exist in manuscript and the last in print, but they also differ in their present materiality for historians. I have seen, read, and picked up the *Pharmacopoeia,* as I have all the other manuscripts I discuss here. I have never seen or held a physical copy of *Florin's Economy,* yet I have read it. In this era of digital copies, the second edition of *Florin's Economy* has been scanned and is available to all as a Google book, on the website and as a downloadable PDF. I was lucky enough to have kind librarians provide me with a PDF of the first edition of *Florin's Economy,* a digitized microfilm of a physical copy. A number of the manuscripts I initially read in the physical original I now also have as JPEGs. If I so choose, I can download those files onto a tablet, open them in a suitable app, then use an electronic pen to annotate them, producing the most up-to-date version of a manuscript gloss. The digital life of pre-modern texts, with all its opportunities and issues, has become vital to historical research, especially as I write this during the COVID-19 pandemic, which has halted so much research with physical materials.[83] Texts, the only extant physical materials of early modern Russian medicine, have now acquired a digital existence that gives them a broader potential audience than mass printing ever did.

Dividing our academic labour into seventeenth and eighteenth century, manuscript and print, makes sense given the necessity for scholars to focus on a limited set of topics on which to be an expert. Yet it can produce unintentional gaps in the secondary literature that are not there in the historical record. The gap between manuscript and print we encounter in histories of medical books in Russia is only a gap of scholarship, not of history. As we see from considering the medical books of the first half of the eighteenth century, the material shift from manuscript to print was a slow, winding river that sometimes doubled back on itself. The material practices of manuscript were gradually marginalized, but never fully destroyed.

CONCLUSION

In order to study long-since-consumed *materia medica* through extant documents, we also need to consider the materiality of the texts that allow us some contact with lost materials of medicine. Looking at Russian medical texts across the late seventeenth and into the eighteenth century, we see several key types of text-as-material. The Apothecary

Chancery relied heavily on manuscript scrolls, long strands of documents to keep the official record. Peter the Great and his successors created decrees and licences in manuscript and print to control medical practice. Private individuals created manuscript medical books. And official institutions printed them. From our position in the present day, we see them through different material eyes, not only as physical scrolls and books, but also as microfilms, PDFs, and JPEGs. Interested as we are in the shifting nature of the materials of early modern official Russian medicine, we then must take account of the material shifts we see in documents about objects, as well as the shifts in objects those documents reveal.

The material paper practices of the seventeenth and eighteenth centuries show us vital aspects of how official Russian medicine functioned. Most vivid is how Latin drafts of reports created for the Apothecary Chancery were folded, and damaged in folding, into the official Russian record. Those Latin drafts collected within them knowledge and opinions taken from many other sources, from both contemporary Western European and ancient Mediterranean world authors, about materials from East Asia to the Americas, the Horn of Africa to the North Sea. Such knowledge was always mobilized to address the questions and fulfill the aims of Russian officialdom, be it understanding a specific kind of *materia medica*, or regulating the use of others. That knowledge was both figuratively and physically subsumed into Russian practices. Tracking the materiality of texts demonstrates how the intertextual practices of early modern Russian medical texts were always subordinate to Russian demands.

The materiality of texts also allows us to build bridges across chasms in our histories of early modern Russian medicine. The printed decrees and books of the eighteenth century look very different from the manuscripts of the seventeenth century. Yet print did not ever really take over from manuscript; the final, printed versions of laws and decrees refer back to earlier legislation in manuscript and were created out of lengthy contemporary considerations that took place in manuscript. Those eighteenth-century processes are a direct continuation of the manuscript practices of the Apothecary Chancery. The printing practices of eighteenth-century Russia, both legal and popular, initially seem different from the manuscript practices of previous centuries. But if we look closely enough at the printed text, we can see the Muscovite manuscript hand that lies beneath.

Conclusion

In 1628 Andrei Loptunov protested his innocence on charges of *maleficia* on the basis of the qualities of the materials with which he was found. In 1748, Fedor Priadunov similarly contested the charges against him for medical malpractice. The former was quietly sent to a monastery, the latter excoriated in a law publicly proclaimed across the entire empire. Yet in a way both shared a common fate. Their practices and their prosecutions were bound up with early modern Russia's particular fixation with consumable medicaments as the major kind of medical practice, and the major site of danger. Walking alongside figures like Loptunov, Priadunov, and their prosecutors allows us to explore the medical world of early modern Russia through the lens of its most central concern: medical drugs.

By the time we begin this book in 1534, with the translation of the *Garden of Health*, Russia already occupied the major part of the Western Eurasian Steppe, stretching from the White Sea in the north to the Black Sea in the south. By the time we end it in 1750, as the Russian government sends out that printed pharmacy decree condemning Priadunov, the decree had to be conveyed from St Petersburg on the Baltic Sea, to Astrakhan on the Caspian, Kyakhta south of lake Baikal in Siberia, and Okhotsk on the Pacific coastline. This sprawling, multi-ethnic, multi-religious empire contained many different doctoring traditions.[1] All of them had to contend with Moscow-based official medicine, embodied in the seventeenth century by the Apothecary Chancery. And that institution cared, above all else, about medical drugs. This was a concern it inherited from the court, and one it shared with other groups in Russian society, notably other parts of the bureaucracy. Yet it was a concern it made its own. Following early modern Russian medicine means, by and large, following drugs.

Like so many other doctoring traditions worldwide, Russia's medical drugs were predominantly plant-based. For Russians, this led to an appreciation of global botanicals. Such a development was not automatic: many doctoring traditions value only local botanicals. For official Russian medicine, however, plants were plants, meaning plants that then only grew many thousands of miles from the Russian Empire were as accepted as the flora of the fields surrounding Moscow. In the sixteenth century, this meant that botanicals from across Afro-Eurasia were combined in the Apothecary Building's mixing bowls. At the start of the seventeenth century, the rising popularity of American botanicals in Afro-Eurasia reached Moscow, and official Russian medicine took full advantage of these new kinds of botanicals for at least the next century and a half. This affection for foreign botanicals is a familiar story, in particular for how it links the history of medicine to the history of colonial violence. Russia has been described by Rachel Koroloff as having its own kind of colonial botany internal to its own empire; examining drugs like sassafras shows that it also benefited from and financially supported the colonial botany of other empires.[2]

In sharp contrast to the prevalence of botanicals, finding chemicals is much harder. They do not appear in the 1580s prescriptions, are almost absent in the first half of the seventeenth century, and only ever make up a minority of medical drug ingredients. The famously taciturn Muscovite official documents do comment on chemicals on occasion, but only to ban them in the 1640s. Yet the medical practitioners at the Russian court, from the 1620s into the eighteenth century, were often vocally pro-chemical medicine. It took them a century to get chemicals accepted into official Russian medicine. More interesting than this outcome is the struggle. It was central and western European medical practitioners, typically Brits, Poles, and Germans, who were pro-chemical; Russian bureaucrats were at best unconvinced of the virtues of chemical medicine. This corresponds with a patterning of chemical medicine elsewhere: it was popular in the German lands and the Ottoman Empire, but suspect in other European nations. Arguments over the value of certain materials took place between communities from different regions and so were, in part, structured geographically.

They were also structured religiously. During the early modern period, many Western Europeans happily used corpse medicine – human remains in consumable medicines. Yet at the start of the seventeenth century, one such medicine, mumia, was declared to be unacceptable to Russian Orthodox Christianity because it was considered unclean. Similarly, theriac, made from vipers' flesh, was also banned. Both bans on flesh-based *materia medica* derived from Russian Orthodox Christianity's strict rules on consumption, limiting certain foods and drinks either periodically or permanently. This decision not to take up two major medicines of the Western European canon takes us to Schiebinger's use of the concept of agnotology, ignorance of something – here, a medicament – because it clashes with cultural values.[3] Eventually, Russians would find a use for fleshy medicines like mumia and theriac, but it would take the major cultural shift of Peter the Great's reign for that to happen. Medical drugs were only accepted to the extent that they fit within society's ideas of human bodies and what they could and should consume.

We have here approached material culture through texts about materials. This is common. Even in cases where we have the objects to examine directly, texts relating to how the object does or should work are key pieces of evidence. Moreover, texts are themselves materials, and are embedded in material practices. The Apothecary Chancery heavily relied upon texts, and had their own textual practices. Key among those practices was the creation of reports: how the department used their experts and texts to produce authoritative statements to answer specific questions for themselves or other departments. When the Apothecary Chancery was closed in the early eighteenth century, these practices lived on. The Academy of Sciences inherited texts from the Apothecary Chancery library; the Medical Chancellery used the same textual practices of investigating and ruling on medical malpractice to help resolve malpractice cases; the Senate then used the conclusions drawn from such cases to revise legislation on pharmacy originally put into place with the help of the Apothecary Chancery. The texts of the Apothecary Chancery have been our specific paper material road to that major kind of medical practice for early modern Russia, the medical drug.

Those specificities take us to generalities. We are here talking about the global history of science and medicine. Ironically, this history has been rather regional, with scholars having to make a significant effort to have their geographic area of study understood as an interconnected part of the early modern global world. It took several years and the focused resolve of a number of scholars to have anglophone histories of early modern global science and medicine recognize Iberia as a major player.[4] Similarly, it has taken the work of historians like Kapil Raj and Pratik Chakrabarti to have the South Asian part of the British Empire acknowledged for its vital role in the science and medicine of that empire.[5] The early modern Russian Empire has never meaningfully been incorporated into the global history of science and medicine. This book shows that Russia was connected to many other world regions, specifically via *materia medica*. When we think globally about early modern science and medicine, we need to include Russia as much as any other major empire. Ignoring the Russian Empire is no longer a viable option.

Global history is disruptive. It can unsettle the geography of early modern global histories by reinserting the Russian Empire where it always should have been. It can also rewrite chronologies. Until now, there has been a very clear timeline of Russian–American relations. The Russian court finds out about the Columbus invasions of the Americas in the sixteenth century; the British try to sell them tobacco in the early seventeenth century but the Russians ban it; the Russians catch sight of the Aleutian Islands in 1732, leading to a creeping colonization centred on what is now called Alaska until its sale to the United States in 1867. Yet turning to *materia medica,* we can see that the Russian elite was keen on American products more than a century before that fateful sighting of the Aleutian Islands. This story disrupts the established history of Russian–American relations by showing a seventeenth-century history never previously considered. It also disrupts the chronology of the Atlantic world, because by expanding the size of the Atlantic world we can see that the Americas were continuously encountered anew by different parts of Eurasia across many decades.

Global history can lead us to local history. Indeed, it is always local concerns that drive global connections. Looking at the specific interest in medical drugs in early modern Russia, which led to the use of African, Asian, and American drugs in Moscow, shows us the importance of this aspect of global connections. If we take literally documents such as the reports with Samuel Collins's name appended to them, we get a history of Western Europeans bringing their expertise to Russia. Yet such a history is flawed, as it obscures both the importance of the Russian elite and the multiple practices of the Russian and non-Russian subjects of the Russian Empire. When Western European medical practitioners provided their expertise, they did so at the behest of the Russian bureaucracy and according to Russian rules, co-constructing official Russian medicine alongside local experts and trying to braid their Western European practices together with local ones.

Those imported experts in the Apothecary Chancery were knowledgeable in any number of subjects, yet what the Russian Empire wanted from them was information on drugs. This local focus on *materia medica* returns us to the vital historiographical question of how to think globally when thinking materially, how to deal with materials when one deals with global history. Historians of science like Chakrabarti and Carla Nappi, and global historians like Anne Gerittsen and Giorgio Riello, have already looked at this problem.[6] This study provides a new perspective, by taking a broad view of an official medical culture specifically invested in *materia medica* but with taboos against certain specific kinds of objects, as shown in the local materials of local texts on global objects. As Nappi, Gerittsen, and Riello have all noted, objects change through time and space, making the study of them tricky. Here, we side-step this issue by taking an unapologetically subjective stance. This book is not a history of global objects, but of one local view of global objects. I cannot tell you everything that theriac was during its global history, but I can tell you how it was viewed in one specific context, the early modern Russian court. One answer to the question of how to deal with global objects is to be local and to take seriously the subjective context in which each object lands. Muscovy shows us how local concerns patterned the global lives of things.

Why include Russia in early modern histories of science and medicine? In part, because it was here all along. Ignoring Russia when writing global histories of early modern science and medicine is to lose a part of that world. But we also need to include the Russian Empire because the Russian context, with its particular focus on the materials of medicine, allows us to more closely examine issues that are hard to make out elsewhere. To look at the meticulous records of the *materia medica* the Apothecary Chancery and Medical Chancellery bought, owned, discussed, examined, prescribed, and banned is to see the huge breadth of choice afforded them. The international contacts and deep pockets of the Moscow court meant the departments could obtain almost anything they wanted. Yet, as it turned out, not everything they could get was something they wanted to have. The best metaphor for the attitude of the early modern Russian elite to the expertise and materials to which they had access are those Latin drafts of the Apothecary Chancery reports, creased and damaged as they were folded into the Russian record. The aim of the court was to extract what they desired from what was available; they had no intention of rewriting their lives by someone else's rules. The story of early modern Russia's fascination with *materia medica* is of the ultimate subjugation of the global to the local.

Appendix One

Ingredients in the *Aptechnaia izba* prescriptions from 1581–1582[1]

Russian name	*English and/or Latin name*	*Kind of material*	*Geographical origin*
Корен торматели	Unidentified	Roots	Unknown
Бет … софеи	Unidentified	Unidentified	Unknown
Попутника большова	Large calla	Flowers	Eurasia
Орешки сканные	Unidentified	Nuts	Unknown
Семени сумак	Sumac seeds	Seeds	Asia/Africa
Коры гранатором	Pomegranate husk	Rind/husk	Asia
Цвет балаустия	Balaustium, wild pomegranate flower	Flower	Asia
Семени барберис	Berberis vulgaris seeds	Seeds	Afro-Eurasia
Семени ситониором	Unidentified	Seeds	Unknown
Тера сизилата	Terra sigillata	Earth	Eurasia
Сок акасия	Acacia sap	Sap	Africa
Сок ипокстидос	Unidentified	Sap	Unknown
Сок таморинги	Tamarind sap	Sap	Africa
Кмину	Cumin	Seeds	Asia
Нукси купреси	Unidentified	Unidentified	Unknown
Мастики	Mastic	Plant resin	Eurasia
Семени петрушкова	Parsley seeds	Seeds	Eurasia
Семени апи	Unidentified	Seeds	Unknown
Семени дауцы	Unidentified	Seeds	Unknown
Сабур	Aloe vera tree	Tree	Middle East
Корен проскурникова большова	Large althaea root	Root	Afro-Eurasia
Семени проскурникова меньшова	Small althaea seeds	Seeds	Afro-Eurasia
Корен девесильный	Inula root	Root	Afro-Eurasia
Корен подлешников	Wild spikenard root	Root	Europe
Есула минор	Unidentified	Unidentified	Unknown

Ingredients in the Aptechnaia izba prescriptions from 1581–1582 – *continued*

Russian name	*English and/or Latin name*	*Kind of material*	*Geographical origin*
Цвет макова	Poppy	Flower	Eurasia
Цвет романова	Chamomile	Flower	Eurasia
Трава мята	Mint	Herb	Eurasia
Трава божей руки	"God's hand"	Herb	Russian Empire
Земляного дым	Fumaria officinalis	Plant	Europe
Прасиум марубиум	Prasium marrubium, white horehound	Plant	Afro-Eurasia
Сена александрина	Alexandrine senna	Leaf	Africa
Ягод вынный	Fig	Fruit	Asia
Диягридиум	Diagridium, from scammony root	Root	Eurasia
Семени проскурникова большова	Large althaea seeds	Seeds	Afro-Eurasia
Баблокакало квинта	Unidentified	Unidentified	Unknown
Масло мятный	Mint oil	Oil	Eurasia
Масло рутный	Ruta oil	Oil	Eurasia
Масло лилиором албором	Lilium album oil	Oil	Eurasia
Патоки белые	White molasses	Syrup	Eurasia
Водка индевеи	Unidentified	Vodka	Eurasia
Водка попутниковы	Calla vodka	Vodka	Eurasia
Корени турбиту	Turpeth root	Root	Asia
Мира булани инди	Myrobalan plum	Fruit	India
Ревень	Rhubarb	Root	Asia
Анис	Anise	Plant	Eurasia
Шефран	Saffron	Plant	Eurasia
Ренское вино	Rhenish wine	Wine	Europe
Спицы Исопи	Unidentified	Plant "needles"	Unknown
Спицы Галанги	Galangal	Plant "needles"	South Asia
Солодкова Дубца	Liquorice stick	Plant	Eurasia

Камедриосу	Teucrium chamaedrys	Plant	Eurasia
Корицы	Cinnamon	Plant	Asia
Инбир	Ginger	Root	Asia
Галгану	Galangal	Root	Asia
Семяни фенюколи	Fennel seeds	Seeds	Eurasia
Семяни карвеи	Unidentified	Seeds	Unknown
Силабалсамум	Unidentified	Unidentified	Unknown
Каменаи	Unidentified	Unidentified	Unknown
Корени перетруну	Pyrethrum	Root	Unknown
Перцу долгова	Long pepper	Plant	Eurasia
Перцу белова	White pepper	Plant	Eurasia
Киприротонда	Unidentified	Unidentified	Unknown
Сквинанте	Squinancywort	Plant	Europe
Корен фьялкова	Iris root	Roots	Eurasia
Семяни амоми	Amomum seeds	Seeds	Asia
Трава подлешник	Wild spikenard	Plant	Europe
Шпико нарды	Unidentified	Unidentified	Unknown
Гумы драганту	Tragacanth	Gum	Middle East
Гумы арабику	Gum arabic	Gum	Africa
Семяни кропова	Dil seeds	Seeds	Eurasia
Семяни зорного	Unidentified	Seeds	Unknown
Иригю	Unidentified	Unidentified	Unknown
Кубебе	Piper cubeba	Plant	Southeast Asia
Гвоздики	Cloves or carnations	Plant	Eurasia
Семяни карпобалсами	Unidentified	Seeds	Unknown
Семяни кардамоми	Cardamom seeds	Seeds	South Asia
Ягоды можжееловые	Juniper berries	Berries	Eurasia
Силерыс мунтаниз	Unidentified	Unidentified	Unknown
Семяни аспорогус	Asparagus seeds	Seeds	Eurasia

Ingredients in the Aptechnaia izba prescriptions from 1581–1582 – *continued*

Russian name	*English and/or Latin name*	*Kind of material*	*Geographical origin*
Корен аспорогус	Asparagus root	Root	Eurasia
Семяни ситри	Citrus seeds	Seeds	Eurasia
Корень акорус	Acorus calamus root	Root	Eurasia
Семяни амиосу	Unidentified	Seeds	Unknown
Орех мушкатные	Nutmeg	Nut	Southeast Asia
Лигном аловес	Lignum aloes	Wood	Southeast Asia
Семяни васильков огородных	Centaurea seeds	Seeds	Eurasia
Корен гарифилата	Garifilata root	Root	Unknown
Семяни воробьева	Unidentified	Seeds	Unknown
Семяни саксыфрагия	Saxifragium seeds	Seeds	Eurasia
Семяни ситроли	Unidentified	Seeds	Unknown
Семяни огуречного	Cucumber seeds	Seeds	Eurasia
Семяни дынного	Melon seeds	Seeds	Eurasia
Семяни арбузного	Watermelon seeds	Seeds	Eurasia
Семяни скарилал	Unidentified	Seeds	Unknown
Маки донского	Don poppy	Plant	Russian Empire
Беналби	Ben albi	Unidentified	Unknown
Бенруби	Ben rubi	Unidentified	Unknown
Стираккаламита	Styrax calamita	Resin	Eurasia
Зерен ячменных	Grains of hordeum	Grain	Afro-Eurasia
Ямидом	Unidentified	Unidentified	Unknown
Сахор головного	Unidentified	Sugar	Unknown
Вода	Water	Water	Local
Итостло електы вариюм дулкус	Unidentified	Unidentified	Unknown
Масла попилиом	Unidentified, could be oil of the popilius eclipticus beetle	Oil	Unknown

Масла своробориннаго	Rose oil	Oil	Eurasia
Водка салатный	“Salad” vodka	Vodka	Unknown
Сироп индивеи	Unidentified	Syrup	Unknown
Оксимелсимъплликс	Oxymel simplex	Honey and vinegar	Eurasia
Водки романовы	Chamomile vodka	Vodka	Eurasia
Корицы маленько	Small cinnamon	Plant	Asia
Семени маку красного	Red poppy seeds	Seeds	Eurasia

NOTE

1 Arranged in order of first appearance in the text. Russian words are given in the nominative but as far as possible the original spelling has been retained, including when certain words have different spellings when they appear in different names. Based on published documents in Zharinov, “Zapisi o raskhode.” I owe much to the work of Kirill Khudin in particular in being able to identify these terms. See for example Khudin, “Nomenklatura lekarstvennykh.”

Appendix Two

Ingredients in Tsar Mikhail Fedorovich's prescriptions from April–June 1645[1]

PRESCRIPTIONS FROM 24 APRIL 1645

Russian name	*English and/or Latin name*	*Kind of material*	*Geographical origin*
Ренское вино	Rhenish wine	Alcohol	Europe
Медведное	Mead	Alcohol	Russian Empire
Эликсир проприэтатис	Elixir proprietatis (made from saffron, aloes, and myrrh)	Compound medicine	Afro-Eurasia
Уха	Fish soup	Animal product	Russian Empire
Безую	Bezoar stone	Animal product	Asia or the Americas
Инроговая кость	Unicorn horn (likely narwhal tusk)	Animal product	North Sea
Соли корольковые	Salt crystals	Salt	Unknown
Зерна перцовые	Peppercorns	Plant	South Asia
Алтеи	Althaea officinalis	Plant	Afro-Eurasia
Кихори	Chicory	Plant	Eurasia
Шкорцинера	Scorzonera	Plant	Eurasia
Полиподии кверцине	Polypodium	Plant	Eurasia
Петрушкое	Parsley	Plant	Eurasia
Ононидисъ всякое	Ononidis of any kind (likely restharrow root)	Root	Europe
Девесильное	Inula	Plant	Afro-Eurasia
Ириосъ	Orris	Plant	Eurasia
Коры капаром	Capparis root bark	Root	Eurasia
Вероника	Veronica	Plant	Eurasia
Агримониа	Agrimonia	Plant	Eurasia
Камедрисъ всякое	Camedris of any kind (likely wall germander)	Plant	Mediterranean

PRESCRIPTIONS FROM 26 MAY 1645

Russian name	*English and/or Latin name*	*Kind of material*	*Geographical origin*
Полынь	Wormwood	Plant	Eurasia
Свороборинное	Rose	Plant	Eurasia
Фьялкое	Iris	Plant	Eurasia
Премери верис	Primula veris	Plant	Eurasia
Гладышевъ	Laserpitium siler	Plant	Europe
ягоды акихенки	Unidentified	Berries	Unknown
Дерева сасафрас	Sassafras wood	Wood	North America
Корица	Cinnamon	Plant	Asia
Гвоздики	Cloves or carnations	Plant	Eurasia
Инбир	Ginger	Root	Asia
Лист александрейскый	Alexandrine senna	Plant	North Africa
Мехиокана чорной	Black michoacán	Plant	Central America
Ревень	Rhubarb	Plant	East Asia
Корен гелебри нигри	Gelebri nigri root (unidentified, possibly a misspelling of gebleri, in which case this is most likely woundwort)	Root	Unknown
Ягоды коринки	Amelanchier berries	Berries	Eurasia OR North America
Кремор татари	Cream of tartar	Acid	Unknown
Расмарина	Rosemary	Plant	Eurasia
Семяни онисового	Aniseed	Plant	Mediterranean
Ягоды можжевеловые	Juniper berries	Berries	Likely Russian Empire
Корен турбиту	Turpeth root	Root	Asia

Мехиокана чорной	Black michoacán	Plant	Central America
Корен турбиту	Turpeth root	Root	Asia
Кремор татари	Cream of tartar	Acid	Unknown
Масло фениколъное	Unidentified oil	Oil	Unknown
Сахар своробоинное	Rose sugar	Sugar	Eurasia
Сахар из цвета розмаринново	Rosemary sugar	Sugar	Eurasia
Сахар из цвета мелиса	Melissa sugar	Sugar	Eurasia esp. Mediterranean region
Сахар из цвета померанцова	Sugar from blood orange	Sugar	Mediterranean region
Коры цытроново	Lemon peel	Rind	South Asia
Конфекси гиацинти	Unidentified	Confectio	Unknown
Магистериумъ из корольковъ красныхъ	Unknown	Unknown	Unknown
Масло коришное	Cinnamon oil	Oil	Asia
Масло гвоздишное	Clove OR carnation oil	Oil	Eurasia
Масло полынюсъ перепускново	Distilled wormwood oil	Oil	Eurasia
Масло купоросное	Vitriol	Acid	Eurasia
Сыроп изъ коры цитроновой	Lemon peel syrup	Syrup	South Asia
Масло мушкатное густова	Thick nutmeg oil	Oil	Southeast Asia
Масла мятное	Mint oil	Oil	Eurasia
Мазь спеленетикомъ	Unidentified	Balm	Unknown
Масло размаринное	Rosemary oil	Oil	Eurasia

PRESCRIPTIONS FROM 5 JUNE 1645

Russian name	*English and/or Latin name*	*Kind of material*	*Geographical origin*
Ладан росное	Incense (type unidentified)	Plant	Asia
Янтар белое	White amber	Amber	Likely Baltic region
Ладан простое	Simple incense	Plant	Asia
Мушкат	Nutmeg	Plant	Southeast Asia

NOTE

1 Arranged in order of first appearance in the text. Multiple uses of one object on the same day have not been noted, but when an object was used on more than one day it has been listed for every day on which it was used. Russian words are given in the nominative but as far as possible the original spelling has been retained, including when certain words have different spellings when they appear in different names. Based on documents published in Mamonov, *Materialy*, 1:120–3; *Akty istoricheskie*, 3:404.

Notes

ABBREVIATIONS

AI	Akty istoricheskie, sobrannye i izdannye arkheograficheskuiu kommissieiu
GIM	Gosudarstvennyi istoricheskii muzei [State Historical Museum, Moscow]
PSZ	Polnoe sobanie zakonov Rossisskoi Imperii
SGGiD	Sobranie gosudarstvennykh gramot i dogovorov, khraniashchikhsia v gosudarstvennoi kollegii inostrannykh del
RGADA	Rossiiskii gosudarstvennyi arkhiv drevnikh aktov [Russian State Archive of Ancient Documents, Moscow]
RGB	Rossiiskaia gosudarstvennaia biblioteka [Russian State Library, Moscow]
RNB	Rossiiskaia natsional'naia biblioteka [Russian National Library, St Petersburg]

INTRODUCTION

1 Chancery Russian, the kind of Russian used in early modern bureaucratic texts, is a term used to distinguish it from the contemporary version of Old Church Slavonic found in religious texts. The two languages are similar but have notable grammatical and semantic differences.

2 Translation from the final Russian version, not Collins's Latin draft, which differs slightly from the final version. All translations are my own

unless otherwise stated. "Елико есть на вселенне наредов, толико есть и жителства отбычает ж, и лекарства вымыслов, и ни един народ озретается тот несмыслен, которой бы, или ненароком, или не отложною никого нуждею принужден честно во употребление лекарства не изобрел бы, что от иных людей скрыто. Бразилиане люди во Америке, наги, и безкнижны, обаче имеет свся лекарства неуничиженна, принесаша бо кам древо сассафрас во употребление, дваяково, яляпии со иными многими изрядных сил израстасмыми. Дивная повествуют хинских дохтурев о искуств, которые без отворениа жил и рожечнаго кровопущаниа тяжча ищия болозни отгоняют, единых ль простым трав своих употреблением, индеяне парами своими отварениа трав со деянными болезни у две прогоняют, а и не намазанми частыми и натиранми которыми блгороднии от рук слуп своих чрез всю идще приемлются, и полегку стискаются, которому делу столь привыкли что без нево усиют не хотят. Могулл великий индейской црь от дохтуров своих еже год наконтарь привышает бы, да оттуду црскаго телесе о прибыли или убыли разсуженье выдам б на часнии дохтуры. и старофавны он у персян обычай, которому приложитися может оное даниила преж црем валтасаром речетое. Аравитяне, хардеи, Греци, Латини, всякие лекарства образцй [здравум разсужением зряще] допущают." RGADA, f. 143, op. 2, ed. khr. 738.

3 Bian, *Know Your Remedies.*

4 Crawford and Gabriel, *Drugs on the Page.*

5 Chipman, *The World of Pharmacy*; Fors, "Medicine and the Making of a City"; Newson, *Making Medicines in Early Colonial Lima;* Shaw and Welch, *Making and Marketing Medicine.*

6 Boumediene, *La colonisation du savoir*; Cook and Walker, "Circulation of Medicine"; Huguet-Termes, "New World Materia Medica in Spanish Renaissance Medicine"; Wallis, "Exotic Drugs and English Medicine."

7 See for example Cook, *Matters of Exchange.*

8 Gänger, "World Trade in Medicinal Plants."

9 Smith, Meyers, and Cook, *Ways of Making and Knowing,* 12.

10 De Laet and Mol, "The Zimbabwe Bush Pump."

11 Clunas, *Superfluous Things.*

12 Nappi, "Surface Tension."

13 Chakrabarti, *Materials and Medicine.*

14 Gerritsen and Riello, *The Global Lives of Things,* 16.

15 Smith, *Entangled Itineraries,* 21.

16 Mukharji, *Doctoring Traditions*, 23.
17 Ibid.
18 Levin, "Healers and Witches in Early Modern Russia."
19 Karoly, *A Turkic Medical Treatise.*
20 Bolsokhoyeva, "Tibetan Medical Schools"; Bolsokhoyeva, "Medical Faculties of Buryat Buddhist Monasteries"; Saxer, "Tibetan Medicine and Russian Modernities."
21 Mukharji, *Doctoring Traditions*, see for example 2–3; Raj, *Relocating Modern Science.*
22 The Apothecary Chancery provided supplies for the creation of holy miro. See Koroloff, "The Patriarchy and the Apothecary." On a man who had lost his mind [обезумел] who was sent to a monastery to recover, see RGADA f. 143, op. 2, ed. khr. 1512.
23 Avvakum Petrov describes taking in the soul-sick in his *Zhitie*; see for example 31. On Archbishop Afanasii of Kholmogory's medical activities, see chapter 3.
24 Shevyrev, "Vvedenie v istoriiu russkoi slovesnosti," 247; Ryan, *Bathhouse*, 72, 85.
25 Kivelson "Political Sorcery."
26 Levin, "Healers and Witches."
27 Dmitrieva, *Povest' o Petre i Fevronii.*
28 Kolesov and Rozhdestvenskaia, *Domostroi*, 15.
29 Emchenko, *Stoglav*, 353.
30 Kivelson, "Political Sorcery."
31 Zagoskin, *Vrachi i vrachebnoe delo*, 19–23. See also Simonov, "Rossiiskie pridvornye matematiki." For general works on pre-modern Russian medicine, see Dörbeck, "Origin of Medicine in Russia"; Liubimenko, "Vrachebnoe i lekarstvennoe delo."
32 Levin, "The Administration of Western Medicine."
33 Griffin, "Povest' preslavna."
34 Griffin, "The Unexotic World."
35 Unkovskaya, *Brief Lives*; Dumschat, *Ausländischer Mediziner.*
36 On foreigners and foreign experts in early modern Russia, see Oparina, *Inozemtsy v Rossii*; Orlenko, *Vykhodtsy iz Zapadnoi Evropy.*
37 Maria Unkovskaya cites a document confirming the existence of the *aptechnaia izba* in 1572: Unkovskaya, "Learning Foreign Mysteries," 5. See also Levin, "The Administration of Western Medicine," 365.
38 Zharinov, "Zapisi o Raskhode."
39 See for example Appleby, "Ivan the Terrible to Peter the Great."
40 On medicine and bureaucracy during the time of troubles, see Liseitsev, "Evoliutsiia prikaznoi sistemy"; Rybalko, *Prikaznaia Biurokratiia*, 22–4.

See also Margeret, *Estat de l'empire,* 53–4; Dunning, *The Russian Empire,* 40.

41 Some Apothecary Chancery documents have been published, notably in Mamonov, *Materialy.* The majority of the archival documents are in the collection RGADA f. 143. Kirill Khudin has done excellent work tracking down documents from the department not included in that collection to their locations in other Russian archives and libraries. See for example Khudin, "Dokumenty aptekarskogo prikaza."

42 For a list of the heads of the Apothecary Chancery, see Liseitsev, Rogozhin, and Eskin, *Prikazy Moskovskogo gosudarstva,* 33–5.

43 On the functioning of the Apothecary Chancery, see in particular Griffin, "Bureaucracy and Knowledge Creation"; Levin, "The Administration of Western Medicine"; Lokhteva, "Materialy Aptekarskogo prikaza"; Sokolovskii, "Kharakter i znachenie."

44 Koroloff, *Seeds of Exchange,* 45–6.

45 Levin, "Administration," 357; Documents of the 10th Nov and 1st Dec 1654 concerning the storage of Apothecary Chancery medicines arrived from Novgorod or the German lands in Rzhev, RGADA f. 143, op. 2, ed. khr. 129.

46 Griffin, "Bureaucracy and Knowledge Creation."

47 Gruzdev, *Russkie rukopisnye travniki,* 25; Unkovskaya, "Learning Foreign Mysteries," 12; Zmeev, *Russkie vrachebniki,* 266.

48 Poe, "Tsar Aleksei Mikhailovich."

49 Demidova, "Buriokratizatsiia gosudarstvennogo apparata" and *Sluzhilaia biurokratiia v Rossii;* Shmidt and Kniaz'kov, *Dokumenty deloproizvodstva,* 9; Utsiugov, "Evoliutsiia prikaznogo stroia." See also Pavlov, "Prikazy i prikaznaia biurokratiia."

50 See chapter 5.

51 Alexander, "Medical Developments in Petrine Russia," 210. See also Haigh, "Design for a Medical Service."

52 The 1721 Senate decree is published in PSZ 6: 412-23. See also Mirskiii, *Meditsina Rossii xvi–xix vekov,* 86.

53 Fond 346 in RGADA. The 1763 decree by Catherine the Great establishing the Medical College is published in Mirskii, *Meditsina Rossii xvi–xix vekov,* 125.

54 Abu-Lughod, *Before European Hegemony.*

55 Green, "Editor's Introduction"; Green, "Taking 'Pandemic' Seriously."

56 Heng, "Early Globalities," 237.

57 Adelman, "What Is Global History Now?"
58 Drayton and Motadel, "Discussion."
59 Charters, Houllemare, and Wilson, *A Global History of Early Modern Violence.*
60 Griffin, "Disentangling Commodity Histories."
61 Flynn and Giráldez, "Globalization Began in 1571."
62 For a recent example of such an approach, see De Zwart and van Zanden, *The Origins of Globalization.*
63 See for example Breen, "Portugal, Early Modern Globalization"; Walker, "The Early Modern Globalization of Indian Medicine."
64 Heng, "Early Globalities," 242–3.
65 De Vries, "The Limits of Globalization."
66 Cooper, "What Is the Concept of Globalization Good For?"
67 Heng, "Early Globalities," 237.
68 Ibid.
69 Ibid.
70 Fan, "The Global Turn."
71 Cañizares-Esguerra, ed., *Entangled Empires.* Raj, *Relocating Modern Science*; Raj, "Beyond Postcolonialism"; Wendt, ed., *The Globalization of Knowledge*; See also Sivasundaram, "Global Histories of Science."
72 Cañizares-Esguerra, *Entangled Empires*, 5.
73 Neilson and Bamyeh, "Drugs in Motion."
74 Breen, "Drugs and Early Modernity," 4. See also Breen, *The Age of Intoxication.*
75 Morozov and Simonov, "Datirovka i atributsiia"; Simonov, *Russkaia astrologicheskaia knizhnost.* On the *Garden of Health* see Bobrova, "Travniki XVI–XVIII vv."; Isachenko, "Travnik Nikolaia Liubchanina"; Isachenko, "Ruskopisi mitropolich'ego skriptoriia"; Isachenko, *Perevodnaia Moskovskaia knizhnost'*; Morozov, "Posleslovie 1616g."; Morozov, "Novoe o travnike"; Morozov, "Vertograd zdraviiu"; Morozov, "K istorii Travnika Liubchanina 1533/34g"; Morozov, "Travnik iz Postel'noi kazny Ivana Groznogo?," Muskala, "K tekstologii."
76 Unkovskaya, *Brief Lives;* Dumschat *Ausländische Mediziner*; Levin, "The Administration of Western Medicine"; Griffin, "Bureaucracy and Knowledge Creation."
77 Dumschat, *Ausländische Mediziner*; Griffin, "Bureaucracy and Knowledge Creation"; Levin, "The Administration of Western Medicine"; Unkovskaya, *Brief Lives.*

78 Graham, *Science in Russia*; Renner, "Wissenschaftstransfer." On eighteenth-century Russian science, see also Gordin, "The Importation of Being Earnest"; Werrett, *Fireworks*; Iosad, "Sciences Strange and Diverse."

79 See for example Arel, "Hospitality at the Hands of the Muscovite Tsar"; Kotilaine, *Russia's Foreign Trade;* Maier and Waugh, "How Well Was Muscovy Connected"; Monahan, *The Merchants of Siberia.*

80 The exception being works on Avraam Petrovich Gannibal, the Russian poet A.S. Pushkin's Russian-African ancestor. See for example Gnammankou, *Abraham Hanibal.*

81 See for example Bolkhovitinov, *Rossiia otkryvaet Ameriky*; Vinkovetsky, *Russian America.*

82 On artisans and early modern science see Smith, *The Body of the Artisan.*

83 Graber et al., "Introduction."

84 Kivelson, *Cartographies of Tsardom*; Kivelson, *Desperate Magic*; Ippolitova, *Russkie rukopisnye travniki;* Lavrov, *Koldovstvo i religiia v Rossii*; Levin, "Healers and Witches"; Smilianskaia, *Volshebniki, bogokhul'niki, eretiki.*

CHAPTER ONE

1 Mukharji, *Doctoring Traditions.*

2 Slater, López-Terrada, and Pardo-Tomás, eds, *Medical Cultures,* 2.

3 Ryan, *Bathhouse,* 269.

4 "Целую сие святое евангелие … не испортить ни которыми делы и ни которою хитростю и зелья лихова и коренья не давати составу нечистаго момии и иного ни какого злаго яду змиина и иных ядовитых зверей и гадов и птиць и всяких злых и ничистих составов которые могут здоровье повредити и испоганить не примешати … над товарыщи своими во всяких составех и вьо всяких мерах которые для их Государского здоровья учнуть составливать смотрети накрепко чтоб они в составех никакого дурна не чинили и зелья лихова вместо добраго." Apothecary Chancery oaths from the reign of Mikhail Fedorovich. Mamonov, *Materialy,* 1:48–9. See also Apothecary Chancery oaths from the reign of Aleksei Mikhailovich, RGADA f. 143, op. 3, ed. khr. 548. Both sets of oaths are markedly similar.

5 Keränen, "The Hippocratic Oath," 59.

6 Dumschat, *Ausländischer Mediziner.*

7 See for example a 1663 report on the venesection of Tsaritsa Mariia Ilinichna in Mamonov, *Materialy,* 2:271–2.

8 Collins's report on venesection, RGADA f. 143, op. 2, ed. khr. 738.

9 Griffin, "Bureaucracy and Knowledge Creation."

10 Apothecary Chancery oaths from the reign of Aleksei Mikhailovich, RGADA f. 143, op. 3, ed. khr. 548.

11 On the directors of the Apothecary Chancery in the context of Muscovite bureaucracy, see Brown, "Military Planning"; Crummey, "The Origins of the Noble Official"; Weickhardt, "Bureaucrats and Boiars."

12 Plavsic, "Seventeenth-Century Chanceries."

13 Unkovskaya, *Brief Lives*, 44.

14 A *dumnyi diak* could earn 530 rubles per annum, a noble 1,450 in official salary before any other entitlements. Hellie, *The Economy and Material Culture*, 416–21.

15 A governor or *stol'nik* could earn 680, an *okol'nichii* 800, a Russian noble 1,450, a foreign expert 2,160, and a general 40,000. Hellie, *The Economy and Material Culture*, 416–21.

16 Here the term "alchemist" denotes someone skilled in the production of complex medicines, through techniques such as distilling, rather than a seeker of the Philosophers' Stone.

17 Unkovskaya, *Brief Lives*, 45–62.

18 An interpreter [*tolmach*] received 100 rubles per annum, a clerk [*podiachii*] 108, a translator [*perevodchik*] 200, and a secretary [*d'iak*] 300. Hellie, *Economy and Material Culture*, 416–21.

19 A smith received 108 rubles per annum, a clerk [*podiachii*] or a *ratnyi chelovek* 150, a *sluzhilyi chelovek* or a secretary [*d'iak*] 300, captain 360. Ibid.

20 Unkovskaya, *Brief Lives*, 64–108.

21 A musketeer [*strelets*] received 66 rubles per annum, a bailiff [*pristav*] 70, a provincial servitor [*gorodovoi dvorianin*] 75, and a sergeant 84. Hellie, *Economy and Material Culture*, 416–21.

22 Unkovskaya, "Foreign Mysteries," 17–18.

23 A guard [*storozh*] received 30 rubles per annum. Hellie, *Economy and Material Culture*, 416–21.

24 Apothecary Chancery oaths from the reign of Mikhail Fedorovich. Mamonov, *Materialy*, 1:48–57.

25 Hulkower, "The History of the Hippocratic Oath," 42.

26 Pelling, "Medical Practice in the Early Modern Period: Trade or Profession?" in *The Common Lot*; Nutton, "What's in an Oath?"; Dorwart, "The Royal College"; Schilling, Schlegelmilch, and Splinter, "Stadtarzt oder Arzt in der Stadt?"; Treue, "Lebensbedingungen jüdischer Ärzte"; Granel "Un serment," 1; Eugène-Humbert, "Les serments professionnels";

Knöpfler, "Eidesformeln für Arzt," 318–20; Wittop Koning, *Compendium*. My thanks to Wouter Klein for his help with the Dutch material.

27 Dorwart, "'The Royal College," 16.

28 Treue, "Lebensbedingungen jüdischer Ärzte," 22–3; Knöpfler, "Eidesformeln," 320–1.

29 Schilling, Schlegelmilch, and Splinter. "Stadtarzt oder Arzt in der Stadt?," 121–3.

30 Dorwart, "The Royal College," 15.

31 Knöpfler, "Eidesformeln für Arzt," 318–20.

32 Treue, "Lebensbedingungen jüdischer Ärzte," 21–3.

33 Wittop Koning, *Compendium*, 46–7.

34 Eugène-Humbert. "Les serments," 122–32.

35 Kivelson, *Desperate Magic*.

36 Kivelson, "Political Sorcery."

37 Discussed in Kleimola, "The Duty to Denounce." See also *AI*, ii, 57; *SGGiD*, ii, 191–4, 202–03, 301–02; *SGGiD*, iii, 14.

38 Kleimola, "Duty to Denounce," 765.

39 Ibid., 764.

40 Clare, "Such a Pretty Tsaritsa."

41 Collis, "Mag elizavetinskoi epokhi"; Simonov, "Rossiiskie pridvornye 'matimatiki'"; on Bomelius see 78–9.

42 Kleimola, "Duty to Denounce," 761.

43 1673 case against Vasilii Likhonin, RGADA f. 143, op. 2, ed. khr. 1054. A 1685 case against Savva Terent'ev and Ganka Fedorov for unlicensed production of spirits, RGADA f. 143, op. 3, ed. khr. 156.

44 A 1685 case against Kuz'ma Dmitriev for replacing essence of rosemary with water, RGADA f. 143, op. 3, ed. khr. 155.

45 RGADA f. 143, op. 2, ed. khr. 1361; Mamonov, *Materialy*, 4:1288–9.

46 Frost, "Prescription and Devotion," 414.

47 A 1703 investigation of Daniel Gurchin, RGADA f. 143, op. 2, ed. khr. 1622.

48 "корень де у него привязан у креста дал ему дорогою идучи прохожий человек и котораго города, того он не ведает, а дал ему тот корень для того, что он Андрейко болен черною болезнью." A 1628 witchcraft investigation against Andrei Loptunov. Novombergskii. *Materialy*, vol. 3, part 1, 9–12. On the meaning of "black illness," see Kolosova, "Name–Text–Ritual," 52.

49 An alternative name for the Apothecary Chancery.

50 "И корень что взять у мужика у Андрейка Лоптунова показован во Аптекарской Палаты дохтурам. И дохтуры Валентин с товарищи смотрев кореня сказали, что тот корень Гусина плоть и к лекарству прогожается, а лихово в нем ничего нет, да и в рот тот корень клали. А будет де кто захочет воровать, и он и на добром корени воровством и наговором дурно сделает, а того де они не знают, ест ли на том корени наговор." Novombergskii, *Materialy*, vol. 3, part 1, 9–12.

51 The term "field herbs" refers to the growing region of those plants as being near to Moscow, and so local.

52 "трава кардиана, другая трава каниса, а те де травы полевые и никакого дурна от тех трав нечает, а иных трав знат не почем, потому что те травы истолчены." A 1664 witchcraft case against Dmitrii Volodemirov, Novombergskii, *Materialy*, 1:60–1.

53 "И в Оптекарском приказе дохтуры и аптекари смотря коренья сказали, что коренье болдерьян и от тово корени ни какова дурна не бывает, а иного коренья им знать не почему, потому что то коренье сухо изгнило и духа никакова от них нет, тако–ж и от тово коренья дурна ни какова нет и из тех кореньев узнали одно коренье и назвали болдерьян а к чему то коренье пригодно – того они не сказали–ж." A 1657 witchcraft trial, Mamonov, *Materialy*, 3:676–7.

54 Culpeper, *The Complete Herbal*, 186–7.

55 Collins's 1665 report on valerian, RGADA f. 143, op. 2, ed. khr. 741; Mamonov, *Materialy*, 3:791–4.

56 A 1657 witchcraft case against Andrei Durbenev. Mamonov, *Materialy*, 3:676–7. A 1664 witchcraft case against syn boyarskii Dmitrii Volodemirov, Novombergskii, *Materialy*, 1:60–01. A 1673 collection of witchcraft cases heard by the Investigations Chancery. Mamonov, *Materialy*, 2:494–5. A 1699 witchcraft case against peasant Mikhail Grigor'ev, RGADA f. 143, op. 3, ed. khr. 454. Witchcraft cases (1703) against Nataliia Elfimova and Ustinia, RGADA f. 143, op. 2, ed. khr. 1618.

57 Novombergskii, *Vrachebnoe stroenie*, XCIII.

58 Levin, "Innocent and Demon-Possessed."

59 A 1652 investigation of Dmitrii Selunskii. Mamonov, *Materialy*, 3:616–18.

60 See for example Pelling and White, *Medical Conflicts*.

61 Zharinov, "Zapisi o raskhode"; see for example recipe no. 7.

62 A 1633 army list. Mamonov, *Materialy*, 1:31–2. Court prescriptions from the 1660s, Mamonov, *Materialy*, 2:278–309.

63 A 1652 investigation of Dmitrii Selunskii, Mamonov. *Materialy*, 3:616–18.

64 Levin, "Healers and Witches," 125–7. On Morozov's tenure in the Apothecary Chancery, see Levin, "Administration," 366–7. This document is conventionally dated to 1662 but Kirill Khudin has shown that this is a mistake in the original document. Khudin, "Lechenie kornem," 390.

65 On such names, see Ippolitova, *Russkie rukopisnye travniki,* 169–206. Khudin has identified this plant as sedum root. Khudin, "Lechenie kornem," 387.

66 A 1662 investigation of Fedor Belozertsov. Novombergskii, *Materialy,* 1:12–13.

67 Khudin, "Lechenie kornem," 392–3.

68 A 1679 malpractice case, RGADA f. 143, op. 2, ed. khr. 1251.

69 A 1685 investigation into the "heady herb," RGADA f. 143, op. 3, ed. khr. 172. On the history of the Kitai-gorod markets selling medicines, see Prussak, "Iz istorii."

70 "в оптеркарскому приказе в оптекарскихъ кн[и]г их нигде не написана чтоб иво внутръ ч[е]л[о]в[е]кому употреблять," RGADA f. 143, op. 3, ed. khr. 172.

71 A 1685 investigation into the "heady herb," RGADA f. 143, op. 3, ed. khr. 172.

72 Oreshnikov, "Danil Gurchin," 47.

73 "внутренних лекарств и иные никаких и масл она Агрофенка не держит." Interrogations of Kitai-gorod market traders (1699), RGADA f. 143, op. 3, ed. khr. 462.

74 On the role of scribes in shaping reported speech in such documents, see Collins, "Speech Reporting"; Collins, *Reanimated Voices.*

75 Fil'kin, "Narodnye apteki."

76 A 1699 investigation into the Kitai-gorod markets RGADA f. 143, op. 3, ed. khr. 462.

CHAPTER TWO

1 Wallis, "Exotic Drugs"; see for example 31–3.

2 Cooper, *Inventing the Indigenous.*

3 Heng, "Early Globalities," 237.

4 Miller, "The Lübeckers"; Bulanin, "Bulev."

5 Isachenko, *Perevodnaia Moskovskaia knizhnost'.*

6 On Daniil's life and works, see for example Bulanin, "Daniil."

7 It is currently thought that a manuscript kept in Kharkiv university library is the 1534 *Garden of Health*. TsNB, 121-r 159/c.

8 The most extensive list of Russian medical manuscripts remains L.F. Zmeev's work. Zmeev, *Russkie vrachebniki*, 5–100.

9 On printed Russian-language medical books in the eighteenth century, see Grombakh, *Russkaia meditsinskaia literature*; Renner, *Russische Autokratie*.

10 Zapasko, *Pam'iatki knizhkovogo mistetstva*, 322; Morozov, "K istorii Travnika Liubchanina"; Morozov, "Travnik iz Postel'noi kazny." It was earlier described in Zhinkin, "Kratkie svedeniia."

11 Bobrova, "Travniki XVI–XVIII vv."; Muskala, "K tekstologii"; Isachenko, "Travnik Nikolaia Liubchanina"; Isachenko, "Ruskopisi mitropolich'ego skriptoriia"; Morozov, "Posleslovie 1616g."; Morozov, "Novoe o travnike"; Morozov, "Vertograd zdraviiu"; Morozov, "K istorii Travnika Liubchanina 1533/34g"; Morozov, "Travnik iz Postel'noi kazny Ivana Groznogo?"

12 See especially Morozov, "Travnik iz Postel'noi kazny Ivana Groznogo?". T.A. Isachenko agrees that this identification is plausible, but also notes that certain aspects of the 1616 manuscript raise some as yet unresolved doubts. Isachenko, *Perevodnaia Moskovskaia knizhnost'*, 153. Johan Muskala states that textological analysis cannot rule out the Kharkiv manuscript as the 1534 protograph but does not consider this identification to be entirely secure. Muskala, "K tekstologii Travnika Liubchanina."

13 Isachenko, *Perevodnaia Moskovskaia knizhnost'*, 135–53; Morozov and Simonov, "Datirovka i atributsiia."

14 RGADA, f. 188, op. 1, ed. khr. 649.

15 Isachenko, *Perevodnaia Moskovskaia knizhnost'*, 153–8.

16 Isachenko, *Perevodnaia Moskovskaia knizhnost'*, 182–93. Published in Florinskii, *Russkie prostonarodnye travniki*, 19–172, and also Isachenko, *Prokhladnyi vertograd*.

17 Isachenko, *Perevodnaia Moskovskaia knizhnost'*, 135–93.

18 Zmeev, *Russkie vrachebniki*, 5–10.

19 N.A. Bogoiavlenskii proposed that the geographic spread of plants in the Slavonic *Garden* was wider, including the American plant sarsaparilla, but the term Bogoiavlenskii identifies as sarsaparilla is *smilax*, which is a genus, not a species. It referred not only to sarsaparilla, but to a number of plants, including china root, which grew in East Asia. Bogoiavlenskii, *Drevnerusskoe vrachevanie*, 48–9. See also Rowell, "Russian Medical Botany," 357. On the usage of the term *smilax*, see Winterbottom, "Of the China Root."

20 Morozov, "Posleslovie 1616g," 133. A 1611 library list from the Kremlin records a *travnik nemetskoi pechati*, proposed by S.A. Belokurov to be the *Gaerde der Sundheit* from which the 1534 translation was made.

21 Morozov, "Posleslovie 1616g," 131–2.

22 Zmeev, *Russkie vrachebniki*, 2–3; Morozov, "Posleslovie 1616g," 132; Zmeev, *Russkie vrachebniki*, 35–52.

23 This can partly be ascertained from what has been proposed about Ivan IV's library. The library no longer exists, and there is some debate as to whether it ever did. See Bogatyrev, "Ivan IV (1533–1584)," 250. For an incomplete list of books kept in Ivan IV's bedchamber, see "Opis' domashnemu," 6–7. For a reconstruction of Ivan IV's library, see Zarubin, *Biblioteka Ivana Groznogo*. For a skeptical view on the existence of Ivan IV's library, see Waugh, "The Unsolved Problem."

24 Morozov has argued it would have been in Ivan IV's personal library, but there is little direct evidence to support such a claim. See in particular Morozov, "Travnik iz Postel'noi kazny Ivana Groznogo?."

25 Morozov, "Novoe o travnike 1616g. (parizhskaia nakhodka)"; Savel'eva, *Katalog knig*, 113–16.

26 Zharinov, "Zapisi o raskhode," 103.

27 Ibid.

28 *Zolotnik* singular, *zolotniki* plural. A *zolotnik* was a common Russian weight used for smaller quantities, and weighed 4.226 grams. Hellie, *The Economy and Material Culture*, 648.

29 My thanks to Emma Spary for her help identifying this item.

30 "Лета 7090-го ноября в 15 день. Дохтор Иван взял про Ивана Яковлича Бельского сена олександрина — 3 золотники, корени турбиту — 4 золотники, мира булани инди — 2 золотника, ревеню — пол 2 золотника; анису, шефрану — по золотнику." Zharinov, "Zapisi o raskhode," recipe no. 5, 123.

31 Andaya, *The World of Maluku*, 2–3.

32 Twelve ingredients are used at least twice. Zharinov, "Zapisi o raskhode," 120–4. On the Maluku Islands in the early modern period, see Andaya, *The World of Maluku*.

33 Isachenko, *Perevodnaia Moskovskaia knizhnost'*, 135–53.

34 TsNB, 121–r 159/c.

35 Griffin, "Bureaucracy and Knowledge Creation."

36 Stone, *A Dictionarie*; Dumschat, *Ausländische Mediziner*, 665–6.

37 Ridley lists 56 disease names and 295 plant names.

38 Stone, *A Dictionarie*, 471–84, 503–17.

39 On the Apothecary Chancery, see Levin, "The Administration"; Dumschat, *Ausländischer Mediziner*. On eighteenth-century Russian medicine see Renner, *Russische Autokratie*; Grombakh, *Russkaia meditsinskaia literatura*.

40 Zharinov, "Zapisi o raskhode," 123.

41 Monahan, "Locating Rhubarb"; Romaniello, "True rhubarb?"; Foust, *Rhubarb*; Burton, *The Bukharans*, 383–5.

42 Monahan, "Locating Rhubarb."

43 Mamonov, *Materialy*, 1:120–3; *AI*, 3:404; Mamonov, *Materialy*, 1:125–7.

44 Collection of prescriptions from 1662, Novombergskii, *Materialy*, 1:1–8. Collection of prescriptions from 1665–1666, RGADA f. 143, op. 2, ed. khr. 743. 1666 prescription RGADA f. 143, op. 2, ed. khr. 745. Collection of prescriptions from 1667–74, Richter, *Geschichte der medicin*, 2:80–7. Collection of prescriptions from 1674 RGADA f. 143, op. 2, ed. khr. 1093. Collection of prescriptions from 1672 Mamonov, *Materialy*, 3:812–14. Supplies sent to establish a pharmacy in Kazan, 1679, Mamonov, *Materialy*, 4:1203–8. Collection of prescriptions from 1698, RGADA f. 143, op. 3 ed. khr. 419.

45 Novombergskii, *Materialy*, 1:49–51.

46 Supplies sent to the army in 1736, RGADA f. 346, op. 1, kn. 9, 328–v. Supplies sent to the army in 1737, RGADA f. 346, op. 1, kn. 9, 329; RGADA 346, op. 1, kn. 3, 752–3; RGADA f. 346, op. 1, kn. 4, 386–r; RGADA 346, op. 1, kn. 4, 548–9; RGADA f. 346, op. 1, kn. 7, 610–11. Supplies sent to Smolensk in 1737, RGADA f. 346, op. 1, kn. 4, 388–9v. Supplies sent to the army in 1749, RGADA f. 346, op. 1, kn. 132, 104v–5; RGADA f. 346, op. 1, kn. 131, 286–v. Supplies sent to the army in 1750, RGADA f. 346, op. 1, kn. 9, 282–3v; RGADA f. 346, op. 1, kn. 132, 437–8v; RGADA f. 346, op. 1, kn. 132, 437–8v; RGADA f. 346, op. 1, kn. 132, 439–40v; RGADA f. 346, op. 1, kn. 132, 411–v; RGADA f. 346, op. 1, kn. 132, 634–v.

47 Zharinov, "Zapisi o raskhode," 123.

48 See in particular Kotilaine, *Russia's Foreign Trade*; Zakharov, *Zapadnoevropeiskie kuptsy*.

49 Fauvelle, *The Golden Rhinoceros*.

50 Martin, *Treasure of the Land of Darkness*, 14.

51 Edwards, "Looking for Abram Hannibal."

52 Mamonov, *Materialy*, 1:120–3; *AI*, 3:404; Mamonov, *Materialy*, 1:125–7.

53 Mamonov, *Materialy*, 3:812–14.

54 Ibid., 709–11, 799–82.

55 Supplies sent to the army in 1737, RGADA f. 346, op. 1, kn. 4, 296–99. Supplies sent to Smolensk in 1737, RGADA f. 346, op. 1, kn. 4, 390–394v. Supplies sent to the army in 1738 RGADA f. 346, op. 1, kn. 4, 419–423. Supplies sent to the army in 1750: RGADA f. 346, op. 1, kn. 9, 209–210.

56 See appendix 1. 1602 import list, Richter, *Geschichte der Medizin*, 1:448–55. 1668 import list, Mamonov, *Materialy*, 2:334–46. 1674 import list, Mamonov, *Materialy*, 2:517–22. 1683 import list, RGADA f. 143, op. 3, ed. khr. 106. 1692 import list, RGADA f. 143, op. 2, ed. khr. 1445. 1694 import list, RGADA f. 143, op. 2, ed. khr. 1513. Collection of prescriptions from 1665, RGADA 143, op. 2, ed. khr. 750.

57 RGADA f. 346, op. 1, kn. 9, 30–1v.

58 Griffin, "Russia and the Medical Drug Trade"; Veluwenkamp and Scheltjens, "Baltic Drugs Traffic."

59 On these trade routes in general, see Nanzatov and Sodnompilova, "Lekarstvennye sredstva." On rhubarb, see Monahan, "Locating Rhubarb"; Romaniello, "True Rhubarb?"; Foust, *Rhubarb*; Burton, *The Bukharans*, 383-85.

60 On Eurasian trade in general, see Burton, *The Bukharans*; Aslanian, *From the Indian Ocean*; Levi, *The Indian Diaspora.* On the trade in medicaments, see Shkunov, "Aptekarskii prikaz"; Nanzatov and Sodnompilova, "Lekarstvennye sredstva."

61 Khudin, "Stanovleniie mozhzhevelovoi povinnosti"; Koroloff, "Juniper."

62 Collection of prescriptions from 1664–65, Mamonov, *Materialy*, 2:278–309. Prescriptions from 1674, ibid., 532–5.

63 1737 document, RGADA f. 346, op. 1, kn. 3, 752–3. 1750 document, RGADA f. 346, op. 1, kn. 9, 209–10.

64 Ippolitova, *Russkie rukopisnye travniki.*

65 See chapter 1.

66 See for example Bolkhovitinov, *Rossiia otkryvaet Ameriky;* Vinkovetsky, *Russian America.* For an overview of historiography on Russian America, see Smith-Peter, "Russian America." I thank Ilya Vinkovetsky for his help on the history of Russian America.

67 Kotilaine, *Russia's Foreign Trade.*

68 Goldstein, "Gastronomic Reforms," 503.

69 Zakharov, *Zapadnoevropeiskie kuptsy*, 200–09, 218–30. I thank Viktor Zakharov for also discussing this topic with me.

70 Romaniello, "Muscovy's Extraordinary Ban."

71 A reference to the old Russian calendar.

72 My thanks to Harold J. Cook for offering this interpretation of what Grek meant by the term "Molikudi."

73 "И древнии убо людие чрезъ Гадиръ плыти не умеяху, паче же не дерзаху; нынешнии же люди португальстии, испанстии, со всякимъ опаствомъ выплываютъ корабли великими, не давно почали, леть тому м, или н, по совершении седмия тысящи, и нашли островов многo, а иныхъ пустыхъ, и землю величайшу глаголемую Куба, еяже конца не ведаютъ тамо живущеи. Нашли же еще, обшедше около всю южскую страну даже до востока солнца зимнаго ко Индии острови семь Молукиди нарицаемыхъ, въ нихъ же родится и корица и гвоздики и ины благовонны ароматы, которыя дотоле не были ведомы ни единому человеческому роду, ныне же всеми ведомы королемъ испанским и португальскимь." Grek, *Sochinenia,* 3:44. Discussed in Bolkhovitinov, *Rossiia otkryvaet Ameriky,* 6–7.

74 Bolkhovitinov, *Rossiia otkryvaet Ameriky,* 6–7.

75 Ibid., 6–7, 229.

76 Boterbloem, *Moderniser of Russia,* 85.

77 See for example, *Vesti-Kuranty, 1656g., 1660–1662g., 1664–1670g. Chast 1,* 128, 514; *Vesti-Kuranty, 1645–46, 1648g,* 164. For a study of translation practices of the *Vesti-Kuranty,* see Maier, "Newspaper Translations."

78 Kivelson's translation. Kivelson, "Between All Parts of the Universe," 170.

79 Ibid.

80 On at least one occasion, the Apothecary Chancery sourced American medicaments from Indian merchants. See Khudin, "Nazvaniia lekarstvennykh."

81 Most likely *C. decidua.*

82 Currently unidentified.

83 *Gvozdiki* can mean cloves or carnations. Here cloves is the more probable translation.

84 Possibly a misspelling of gebleri, in which case this is most likely woundwort.

85 "Коренъя: Алтеи 6 золотниковъ. Кихори. Шкорцинера. Полиподии кверцине. Петрушкого. Ононидисъ всякого по 3 золотники. Девисильного. Ириось по 2 золотника. Коры капаромъ 6 золотниковъ.

Травы: Вероника. Агримониа. Камедрисъ всякого по горсти. Полынью 2 щепотки.

Цветы: Свороборинного. Фьялкого по 2 щепотки. Примери верисъ. Гладышевъ по щепотьке. Ягодъ акихенки 3 золотника. Дерева сасафрау 3 золотника. Корицы 3 золотника. Гвоздики полъ 2 золотника. Инбирю 2 золотника. Листу александрейскаго 12 золотниковъ. Мехиокана чорной. Ревеню по 3 золотники. Кореню гелебри нигри полъ золотника. Ягодъ коринки 12 золотниковъ креморъ тартари 2 золотника. Размарину щепотка. Семяни онисового 3 золотника. Ягодъ мозжевеловыхъ 6 золотниковъ.

Вино ренское составлено съ разными травы и коренья." Mamonov, *Materialy*, 1:120–3; *AI*, 3:404.

86 Stone, *A Dictionarie*; Annenkov, *Botanicheskii slovar'*; Utkin, *Kratkii botanicheskii.*

87 Karoly, *A Turkic Medical Treatise.*

88 Koroloff, *Seeds of Exchange*, 40–1.

89 Griffin, "Disentangling Commodity Histories."

90 Bleichmar, "Books, Bodies, and Fields," 88.

91 Ibid., 96.

92 Griffin, "Disentangling Commodity Histories."

93 Mamonov, *Materialy*, 1:120–3; *AI*, 3:404.

94 Crellin, "Early Settlements."

95 Romaniello, "Humoral Bodies."

96 1602 import list, Richter, *Geschichte der Medizin*, 1:448–55. 1633 list of supplies for the army, Mamonov, *Materialy*, 1:31–2.

97 On sassafras use see Mamonov, *Materialy*, 2:278–309; on the use of Michoacán root see Richter, *Geschichte der Medizin*, 2:93, and also the use of jalap, 2:80–87.

98 Ibid., 2:94

99 Stephenson, "From Marvelous Antidote."

100 Mamonov, *Materialy*, 4:1294–1300.

101 RGADA f. 143, op. 3, ed. khr. 419.

102 RGADA f. 143, op. 3, ed. khr. 419.

103 Winterbottom, "Of the China Root"; Borschberg, "The Euro-Asian Trade."

104 RGADA f. 346, op. 1, kn. 7, 585–v; RGADA f. 346, op. 1, kn. 7, 585–v; RGADA f. 346, op. 1, kn. 9, 350–3; RGADA f. 346, op. 1, kn. 7, 588–v; RGADA f. 346, op. 1, kn. 9, 30–1v; RGADA f. 346, op. 1, kn. 9, 32–3. On Peruvian balsam see Maehle, *Drugs on Trial*, 224.

105 On jalap: RGADA f. 346, op. 1, kn. 3, 342–3; RGADA f. 346, op. 1, kn. 9,

300–v; RGADA f. 346, op. 1, kn. 9, 350–3; RGADA f. 346, op. 1, kn. 9, 30–1v; RGADA f. 346, op. 1, kn. 9, 32–3; RGADA f. 346, op. 1, kn. 9, 323–v. On sassafras and sarsaparilla: RGADA f. 346, op. 1, kn. 9, 350–3; RGADA f. 346, op. 1, kn. 7, 591; RGADA f. 346, op. 1, kn. 7, 588–v; RGADA f. 346, op. 1, kn. 7, 439–56v.

106 RGADA f. 346, op. 1, kn. 131, 14; RGADA f. 346, op. 1, kn. 132, 568–70. On ipecancuanha, see Gänger, "World Trade," 45.

107 Griffin, "Disentangling Commodity Histories," 16.

108 In 1597, the Republic of Venice was offered the chance to buy a unicorn horn at the price of 30,000 ducats. Given the current price of gold at around 60USD a gram (as of December 2021) and that a ducat was around 3.5 grams of gold, this is around 6,300,000USD for the horn. This was almost certainly a narwhal tusk, which can weigh up to 10 kilos, making for an approximate per kilo price of 3,000 ducats or 630,000USD. Shepard, *Lore of the Unicorn*, 108.

109 See for example prescriptions from 1664–65 where sassafras was prescribed in quantities of between 0.5 and 12 *zolotniki*. Mamonov, *Materialy*, 2:278–309.

110 Griffin, "Russia and the Medical Drug Trade," 16.

111 Stadsarchief Amsterdam, collection no. 6, documents 97, 98. Collection no. 78, documents 399, 404, 414.

112 Veluwenkamp and Scheltjens, "Baltic Drugs Traffic."

113 *Florinova Ekonomiia* (1738), 288; *Florinova Ekonomiia* (1760), 325.

114 Chakrabarti, "Empire and Alternatives."

115 Monahan, "Locating Rhubarb."

116 Koroloff, "In imperio Rutheno."

117 Heng, "Early Globalities," 237.

CHAPTER THREE

1 Simioli, "The King of Essences"; McVaugh, "Chemical Medicine"; Trambaiolo, "Antisyphilitic Mercury"; Bian, *Know Your Remedies*.

2 Mendoza and Wolter, "Medicine in Meso and South America," 2.

3 Hedesan, "Alchemy, Potency, Imagination"; in particular 93–4.

4 Porter *The Greatest Benefit*, 201–10.

5 De Vos, "From Herbs to Alchemy"; Shefer-Mossensohn, *Ottoman Medicine*, 177; Moran, "A Survey of Chemical Medicine"; Savage-Smith, "Drug Therapy of Eye Diseases"; Küçük, "Medical Translations."

6 For an interpretation of this as chemical medicine, see de Madariaga, *Ivan the Terrible,* 351–6; Bogatyrev, "Ivan IV (1533–1584)," 252. For a contrary view that argues there was no alchemy or chemical medicine in Russia before 1600, see Figurovskii, "The History of Chemistry." On the autopsies, see Panova, *Kremlevskie usypal'nitsy,* 214–18; Babichenko, "Kremlevskie tainy"; Gerasimov, "Dokumental'nyi portret" and "Portrety istoricheskikh lits"; Kobrin, *Ivan Groznyi,* 132–3; Skrynnikov, *Tsarstvo terrora,* 501; Crummey, *The Formation of Muscovy 1304–1613,* 143–5, 162–3, 173; Hellie, "In Search of Ivan the Terrible," xxxiv; Keenan, "Vita: Ivan Vasil'evich," 48–9 and "Ivan IV and the 'King's Evil'"; Keenan and Martin, "The Tsar's Two Bodies"; Prozorovskii and Kolosova, "Nekotorye dannye"; Prozorovskii, Alisievich, Kanter, and Rubtsov, "Issledovanie ostatkov tsaria Ivana IV." I thank the numerous scholars of H-EarlySlavic who contributed to a series of interconnected threads on the autopsies in 2001–02.

7 Ryan, "Alchemy, Magic, Poisons"; Ryan, "The Old Russian Version"; Ryan, "The *Secretum Secretorum*"; "Alchemy and the Virtues of Stones."

8 See chapter 2.

9 Apothecary Chancery oaths from the reign of Aleksei Mikhailovich, RGADA f. 143, op. 3, ed. khr. 548.

10 Raj, *Relocating Modern Science.*

11 Pareja, *Confessionario*; Dubcovsky and Broadwell, "Writing Timucua."

12 Shapin, "The Invisible Technician."

13 Richter, *Geschichte der medicin,* 2:12–22.

14 Newman and Principe, *Alchemy Tried in the Fire.*

15 See for example French, *John Dee.*

16 Unkovskaia, *Brief Lives,* 9–10; Dumschat, *Ausländischer Mediziner,* 591–4; Figurovski, "The Alchemist and Physician."

17 Abraham, "The Sources."

18 See for example Dee, *Fasciculus chemicus,* 149–50. Comments here are based on the 1644 Latin edition as this was the earliest edition available with a specific date of publication indicated.

19 "Opera & studio Arthuri Dee, Archiatri Magni Imperatoru totius Russiae." Dee, *Fasciculus chemicus,* 1. On Gurchin's references to his courtly associations, see chapter 5.

20 See chapter 5.

21 Apothecary Chancery oaths from the reign of Aleksei Mikhailovich, RGADA f. 143, op. 3, ed. khr. 548.

22 Debus, *The Chemical Philosophy*, 190.

23 1602 import list Richter, *Geschichte der medicin*, 1:445.

24 Karpenko and Norris, "Vitriol"; Debus, *The French Paracelsians*, 36, 77, 198.

25 1645 import list from Hamburg. Mamonov, *Materialy*, 1:79–86. 1647 import list from Amsterdam. Mamonov, *Materialy*, 3:601–04.

26 Mamonov, *Materialy*, 1:2; Mamonov *Materialy*, 1:3; Mamonov, *Materialy*, 1:4; Mamonov, *Materialy*, 1:11; Mamonov, *Materialy*, 1:14-15; Mamonov, *Materialy*, 1:16; Mamonov, *Materialy*, 1:19; Mamonov, *Materialy*, 1:38; Mamonov, *Materialy*, 1:38; Mamonov, *Materialy*, 1:39. 1633 prescription for Vasilii Streshnev including vitriol, *AI*, 3:473.

27 Mamonov, *Materialy*, 1:41–3; *AI*, 3:386; Mamonov, *Materialy*, 1:48; Mamonov, *Materialy*, 1:58; Mamonov, *Materialy*, 1:120–3; *AI*, 3:404; Mamonov, *Materialy*, 1:124; *AI*, 3:479; Mamonov, *Materialy*, 1:124; Mamonov, *Materialy*, 1:124–5; Mamonov, *Materialy*, 1:125; Mamonov, *Materialy*, 1:125–7; *AI*, 3:471–2.

28 Mamonov, *Materialy*, 3:599–600; Mamonov, *Materialy*, 3:610–11.

29 Debus, *The French Paracelsians*, 21.

30 Those including vitriol are published in Mamonov, *Materialy*, 1:32–3 and 35–7; *AI*, 3:473 and 474.

31 The prescription including the plaster stiptikum is *AI*, 3:473.

32 John Woodall included it in his popular naval medical text *The Surgions Mate* in 1617. Interestingly, the mentions Woodall makes to the Paracelsus plaster seem to assume a familiarity with that item on the part of the reader, suggesting it was a well-known part of medicine in this period. Woodall, *The Surgions Mate*, 136, 138.

33 Quincy, *Pharmacopoeia Officinalis*, 469.

34 1644 list of provisions sent to Count Valdemar of Denmark to treat his horses, including vitriol, Mamonov, *Materialy*, 1:124. 1645 prescription including the Paracelsus plaster, Mamonov, *Materialy*, 1:58. 1647 request for treatment by servitor including vitriol, Mamonov, *Materialy*, 3:599-600. Undated prescription to Tsaritsa Maria Ilichna, including vitriol, Mamonov, *Materialy*, 3:606-7. 1648 request for medical supplies to treat the Danish Ambassador's son, including vitriol, Paracelsus plaster and antimony, Mamonov, *Materialy*, 3:610-11.

35 Pelling and White, *Medical Conflicts*; Debus, *The French Paracelsians*; Rankin, "Empirics, Physicians, and Wonder Drugs."

36 Panova, *Kremlevskie usypal'nitsy*, 214–18; Babichenko, "Kremlevskie tainy"; Gerasimov, "Dokumental'nyi portret" and "Portrety istoricheskikh lits"; Kobrin, *Ivan Groznyi*, 132–3; Skrynnikov, *Tsarstvo terrora*, 501; Crummey, *The Formation of Muscovy 1304–1613*, 143–5, 162–3, 173; Hellie, "In Search of Ivan the Terrible," xxxiv; Keenan, "Vita: Ivan Vasil'evich," 48–9 and "Ivan IV and the 'King's Evil'"; Keenan and Martin, "The Tsar's Two Bodies"; Prozorovskii and Kolosova, "Nekotorye dannye"; Prozorovskii, Alisievich, Kanter, and Rubtsov, "Issledovanie ostatkov tsaria Ivana IV."

37 Grell, Cunningham, and Arrizabalaga, *It All Depends on the Dose*; Parascandola, *King of Poisons*.

38 RGADA f. 143, op. 1, ed. khr. 1a.

39 Richter, *Geschichte der medicin*, 2:80–7.

40 Richter, *Geschichte der medicin*, 2:87–92.

41 Mamonov, *Materialy*, 3:1294–300.

42 Richter, *Geschichte*, 2:80–7.

43 Mamonov, *Materialy*, 4:1294–300.

44 RGADA f. 143 op. 3 ed. khr. 419.

45 RGADA f. 143, op. 2, ed. khr. 306; Mamonov, *Materialy*, 3:696.

46 Richter, *Geschichte der medicin*, 2:80–7.

47 Mamonov, *Materialy*, 4:1294–1300.

48 RGADA f. 143, op. 3, ed. khr. 419.

49 Panich, *Literaturnoe tvorchestvo*, 124–5. Panich partly follows A. Viktorov, who argued that Gurchin helped Afanasii of Kholmogory compile this text. Viktorov, *Sobranie slaviano-russkikh rukopisei*, 28.

50 Burke, "Cultures of Translation," 31–3.

51 "Формокопиа о составлении лекарствъ переведенная с латынского языка на словенский от р[о]ж[д]ества христова 1676," RGB f. 37, no. 228, 7.

52 Panich, *Literaturnoe tvorchestvo*, 131.

53 RGB f. 37, no. 228.

54 Unkovskaya, *Brief Lives*, 53–4.

55 "Спиритус салисъ армоняцы составливается онъ сице.
Нашатырю извести купоросу красного з женом воды свежей чистой смешать вместе и поставить на двои или на трои сутки заткнувъ в склянке и после взмутить в другую склянку сквозь серую бумагу начисто, и беречь заткуть склянку крепко. а нюхать ево от главныя болезни и от залегания ноздрей." RGB f. 37, no. 228, 41v–42r.

56 RGB f. 37, no. 228, 41v and 42r–v. Also known as Daniel (von) Gaden. Stefan was the name he was baptized with when he converted to Russian Orthodox Christianity. Unkovskaya, *Brief Lives*, 34–7.

57 Savel'eva, *Katalog knig.*

58 Florinskii, *Russkie prostonarodnye travniki*, 19–172, and Isachenko, *Prokhladnyi vertograd.*

59 1672 translation of a German medical book, Zmeev, *Vrachebniki*, 72–3. 1679 ten medical books ordered to be translated, RGADA f. 143, d. 2, ed. khr. 1290. On Latin-Russian translation of medical texts and terms, see Leeming, "Polish and Polish-Latin."

60 Schröder, *Pharmocopoeia medicochymica*, RGADA f. 143, op. 2, ed. khr. 903. Hortius, *Pharmacopoiea Galeno-Chemica.* Savel'eva, *Katalog knig*, 93–4. It is also mentioned in an early eighteenth-century list of works held by the Medical Chancellery, the Apothecary Chancery's successor. See Khoteev, "Biblioteka Leib-medika," 44–7.

61 Levin, "Administration," 371–2; RGADA f. 143, op. 3, ed. khr. 536.

62 1690 report on graduates of Padua university, RGADA f. 143, op. 3, ed. khr. 322.

63 "Тело же убо человече от четырь състав, глаголем, съдано. Имать бо от огня теплоты, от възвуха же студеньство, от земля же сухоту, от воды же мокроту." Mil'kov, "Antichnoe uchenie," 60.

64 "Миръ от че(ты)рех вещеи състави(с). От огня. От вздоуха. От земля. И от воды," Mil'kov, "Antichnoe uchenie," 59.

65 "Яко таких которым во Италии огнь и вод им не подается, что глубее естества сокровенная истязают, и самое преизрядное учение тиснение не одному токмо Парацелсу или Хелмонцию но и великому Иппократу Платону и иным предревним учителем и которым ныне не отдавных принимают и почитают." RGADA f. 143, op. 3, ed. khr. 322.

66 Dooley, "Social Control," 229.

67 Clericuzio, "From van Helmont to Boyle," 304.

68 Pantin, "The Role of Translations," 172.

69 Tsvetaev, *Mediki v Moskovskoi Rossii*, 23–7.

70 Hughes, *Russia*, 305–06.

71 Koroloff, "The Patriarch and the Apothecary."

72 Panich, *Literaturnoe tvorchestvo*, 125–6.

73 Ibid., 124–6, 130–3.

74 Ibid., 191–206.

75 “Состав мази свербежной счинить так.
Взять девесилу свежево, да луку, сколько хочешь, истолочь вместе, и положить в масло коровье, чтоб масло против лука было половина, и девесила придать, соли, горсть, серы горячей толченой горсть. И сварить вместе, дондеже сырость выкипит, а со огня сняв, и выжать скрозь плат на блюдо древяное или в ставец. И тот состав приложить рдути [так], и смешать, дондеже ртуть замрет, а мазь преисинеет. И тою мазию намазывать свербежные места – зело сушит и живит.” Panich, *Literaturnoe tvorchestvo*, 200–01.

76 The exact roles of Blumentrost and Gurchin in the creation of the *Domestic and Field Pharmacy* are disputed, as is the text’s relationship both to Blumentrost’s earlier *Pharmacotheca domestica et portatilis* and to his later 1715 *Haus und Reise Apotheke*. See Prussak, “Obzor meditsinskikh rukopisei,” 24–5; Sokolovskii, “Kharakter i znachenie,” 85; Griffin, “In Search of an Audience” and “The Production and Consumption,” 164–7.

77 GIM Uvar., no. 172, 5v.

78 “я химическую и аптекарскую науку из младыхъ лету всегда чтился,” GIM Uvar., no. 172, 1–2v.

79 Griffin, “In Search of an Audience.”

80 BAN, Petrine collection, no. 75.

81 RNB, Pogodin collection, no. 1561, l. 116v.

82 RNB, f. 550, O., VI., 4.

83 RNB, f. 550, O., VI., no. 12, recipe number 16.

84 See 1737 RGADA f. 346, op. 1, kn. 9, 103–v. 1737 RGADA f. 346, op. 1, kn. 7, 585–v. 1737 RGADA f. 346, op. 1, kn. 7, 591. 1737 RGADA f. 346, op. 1, kn. 7, 583–584v. 1750 RGADA f. 346, op. 1, kn. 132, 308. 1750 RGADA f. 346, op. 1, kn. 132, 291–v.

85 1737 RGADA f. 346, op. 1, kn. 9, 67–8. 1737 RGADA f. 346, op. 1, kn. 9, 350–3. 1737 RGADA f. 346, op. 1, kn. 7, 591. 1737 RGADA f. 346, op. 1, kn. 9, 32–3. 1738 RGADA f. 346, op. 1, kn. 7, 439-456v. 1750 RGADA f. 346, op. 1, kn. 132, 568–70.

86 RGADA f. 346, op. 1, kn. 7, 439–56v.

87 Records from 1737: RGADA f. 346, op. 1, kn. 3, 752-53; RGADA f. 346, op. 1, kn. 4, 257-69; RGADA f. 346, op. 1, kn. 9, 155–v; RGADA f. 346, op. 1, kn. 4, 296–9; RGADA f. 346, op. 1, kn. 4, 307–08; RGADA f. 346, op. 1, kn. 4, 386–r; RGADA f. 346, op. 1, kn. 4, 388–9v; RGADA f. 346, op. 1, kn. 4, 508–09; RGADA f. 346, op. 1, kn. 7, 495–6; RGADA f. 346, op. 1, kn. 7,

497–9; RGADA f. 346, op. 1, kn. 7, 610–11. Records from 1749: RGADA f. 346, op. 1, kn. 132, 104–v; RGADA f. 346, op. 1, kn. 132, 104v–105. Records from 1750: RGADA f. 346, op. 1, kn. 9, 209–10; RGADA f. 346, op. 1, kn. 132, 437–8v; RGADA f. 346, op. 1, kn. 132, 439–40v; RGADA f. 346, op. 1, kn. 132, 411–v; RGADA f. 346, op. 1, kn. 132, 634–v; RGADA f. 346, op. 1, kn. 131, 333–5.

88 Mikhailov, *Meditsinskaia sluzhba russkogo flota,* 128–9.

CHAPTER FOUR

1 For example, Spanish conquistadors worried that their bodies would take on non-European aspects through consuming American products. Earle, *The Body of the Conquistador.*

2 Schiebinger, "Feminist History."

3 Nabil Matar has shown how coffee was associated with Islam in early modern Britain and so seen as a threat to a European drinkers' Christianity. Matar, *Islam in Britain,* 115–19.

4 Boumediene, *La colonisation du Savoir.*

5 Norton, *Sacred Gifts*; Norton, "Tasting Empire."

6 Akasoy and Yoeli-Tlalim, "Along the Musk Routes."

7 Fabbri, "Treating Medieval Plague"; Nappi, "Bolatu's Pharmacy Theriac."

8 Nappi, "Bolatu's Pharmacy Theriac"; Beckwith, "Tibetan Treacle."

9 Dannenfeldt, "Egypt and Egyptian Antiquities," 17.

10 Apothecary Chancery oaths from the reign of Mikhail Fedorovich. Mamonov, *Materialy* 1:48. See chapter 1.

11 Although the Apothecary Chancery did on occasion prescribe medicines for high-status animals, in particular, horses kept at court, the department was primarily dedicated to treating humans. On prescriptions for horses see for example Mamonov, *Materialy* 1:124.

12 Herzberg, "Faith on the Menu," 386. See also Stenfors and Hellie, "The Elite Clergy Diet."

13 Goldstein, "Gastronomic Reforms," 485.

14 Herzberg, "Faith on the Menu," 390.

15 Brostrom, *Archpriest Avvakum,* 65–6; Petrov, *Zhitie,* 30–1.

16 Berry and Crummey, *Rude and Barbarous Kingdom,* 228.

17 Poe, *Samuel Collins. The Present State of Russia,* 19.

18 Herzberg, "Faith on the Menu," 393; Dumschat, *Ausländische Mediziner,* 298–9.

19 Ibid., 395–7.

20 Thyrêt, "'Blessed Is the Tsaritsa's Womb'"; Griffin, "Such a Pretty Tsaritsa."
21 Herzberg, "Faith on the Menu," 390.
22 Kaiser, *Death and Dying*, 18–20.
23 Levin, "Supplicatory Prayers."
24 A 1644 post-mortem of a member of Prince Valdemar of Denmark's retinue. Mamonov, *Materialy*, 1:62–3.
25 Unkovskaya, "Foreign Mysteries," 10; Mamonov, *Materialy*, 3:727–8.
26 On saints' bodies in Western Europe, see Geary, "Sacred Commodities"; de Ceglia, "Thinking with the Saint." On saints in early modern Russia see Lenhoff, "The Notion of 'Uncorrupted Relics'"; Levin, "From Corpse to Cult"; Levin, "Innocent and Demon-Possessed."
27 Park, "The Life of the Corpse."
28 Lenhoff, "The Notion of 'Uncorrupted Relics.'"
29 Apothecary Chancery oaths from the reign of Mikhail Fedorovich. Mamonov, *Materialy*, 1:48. See chapter 1.
30 Here I am following the spelling used by Dannenfeldt. See for example Dannenfeldt, "Egyptian Mumia."
31 Dannenfeldt, "Egypt and Egyptian Antiquities," 17.
32 Dannenfeldt, "Egyptian Mumia"; Siraisi, *History*, 229–30; Park, "The Life of the Corpse"; Sugg, "'Good Physic'"; Sugg, *Mummies, Cannibals*; Schmitz-Esser, *Der Leichnam im Mittelalter*. I am grateful to Albrecht Classen for the reference to Schmitz-Esser's work.
33 Dannenfeldt, "Egypt and Egyptian Antiquities," 19.
34 Park, "The Life of the Corpse," 116.
35 Dannenfeldt, "Egyptian Mumia," 173.
36 Nappi, "Bolatu's Pharmacy Theriac," 739.
37 Heaney, "How to Make an Inca Mummy," 13.
38 Cooper, *Inventing the Indigenous*.
39 Dannenfeldt, "Egypt and Egyptian Antiquities," 21.
40 Mamonov, *Materialy*, 1:48.
41 A 1645 import from Hamburg. Mamonov, *Materialy*, 1:79–86. A 1646 import from Amsterdam. Mamonov, *Materialy*, 3:601–04. A 1660 import from unknown location. Novombergskii, *Materialy*, 1:9–10. A 1667 import from Hamburg. Mamonov, *Materialy*, 2:334–46. A 1629 prescription. Mamonov, *Materialy*, 1:2. A 1629 prescription, Mamonov, *Materialy*, 1:3. 1630 prescription, Mamonov, *Materialy*, 1:4. A 1630 prescription, Mamonov, *Materialy*, 1:11. A 1631 prescription, Mamonov, *Materialy*, 1:14–15. A 1631 prescription, Mamonov, *Materialy*, 1:16. A

1631 prescription, Mamonov, *Materialy*, 1:19. A 1633 prescription, Mamonov, *Materialy*, 1:38. A 1633 prescription, Mamonov, *Materialy*, 1:39. A 1643 prescription, Mamonov, *Materialy*, 1:41–3. A 1643 prescription, Mamonov, *Materialy*, 1:48. A 1644 prescription, Mamonov, *Materialy*, 1:124. A 1644 prescription, Mamonov, *Materialy*, 1:124. A 1644 prescription, Mamonov, *Materialy*, 1:124–5. A 1645 prescription, Mamonov, *Materialy*, 1:120–3. A 1645 prescription, Mamonov, *Materialy*, 1:125. A 1645 prescription, Mamonov, *Materialy*, 1:125–7. A collection of prescriptions from 1629–45, *AI*, 3:471–2.

42 My translation is of the Russian version; I have been unable to track down the original. "Дьявольская резня продолжалась с 3 часов до 11. Поляков погибло 2135; в числе убитых были студенты, Немецкие ювелиры и купцы Аугсбургские, имевшие много денег и всякого добра. Злодеи бросали тела убиенных на улицы, в жертву собакам и Русским площадным лекарям, которые вырезали жир из трупов. Двое суток лежали мертвые под открытым небом; в третий день убийца Шуйский приказал их подобрать и похоронить в Божьем доме." http://www.vostlit.info/Texts/rus10/Ber/frametext2.htm (accessed 16 June 2021). My thanks to Alexei Lobin for pointing me to the original source of this comment, which I had only previously seen repeated without citation in Zmeev, *Russkie vrachebniki*, 109. For an account of Bäer's time in Moscow and his courtly connections, see Tsvataev, *Protestantskie tserkvi*, 33–4.

43 Davies and Matteoni, "'A Virtue beyond All Medicine,'" 701.

44 For a history of this period, see for example Dunning, *Russia's First Civil War*.

45 Zmeev, *Russkie vrachebniki*, 109.

46 Rowland, "The Problem of Advice," 270.

47 Liseitsev, *Posol'skii prikaz*; Liseitsev, "Evoliutsiia prikaznoi sistemy"; Rybalko, *Rossiiskaia prikaznaia biurokratiia*.

48 Mamonov, *Materialy*, 1:48. See chapter 1.

49 "Ils ne sçavent que c'est de Medecines, si ce n'est l'Empereur et quelques principaux Seigneurs. Mesmes ils tiennent plusieurs choses souillées, desquelles on se sert en Medecine, entr'autres ne prennent volontiers des Pilules. Quant aux Clisteres, ils les abhorrent, comme aussi le Musc, la Civete, et autres telles choses. Mais si les simples sont malades, ils prennent coustumiere ment un bon traict d'eau de vie, et y mettent une charge de poudre d'arquebouze dedans, ou bien une teste d'ail pilée,

remuent cela et le boi vent, et vont à l'instant a une estuve, laquelle est si chaude, que l'on n'y sçauroit presque durer, et y demeu rent iusques à ce qu'ils ayent sué vne heure ou deux, et en usent de mesme en toute sorte de maladies." Margeret, *Estat de l'empire,* 53–4. For an English translation of Margeret's account, see Dunning, *The Russian Empire,* 40.

50 Akasoy and Yoeli-Tlalim, "Along the Musk Routes."

51 In the early modern period this was a synonym for theriac; only later did it take on its meaning of a sweet syrup.

52 Poe, *Samuel Collins. The Present State of Russia,* 19.

53 Prescriptions from 1629. Mamonov, *Materialy,* 1:2–3; 1630 prescriptions. Mamonov, *Materialy,* 1:4, 11; 1631 prescriptions, Mamonov, *Materialy,* 1:14–16, 19; 1633 prescriptions, Mamonov, *Materialy,* 1:38–9; 1643 prescriptions, Mamonov, *Materialy,* 1:41–3, 48; *AI,* 3:386; 1644 prescriptions, Mamonov, *Materialy,* 1:124–5; *AI,* 3:479; 1645 prescriptions, Mamonov, *Materialy,* 1:120–3, 125–7; *AI,* 3:404; collection of prescriptions from 1629–45, *AI,* 3:471–2.

54 A 1602 import list, Richter, *Geschichte,* 1:448–55; 1645 import list, Mamonov, *Materialy,* 1:79–86; 1647 import list, Mamonov, *Materialy,* 3:601–04.

55 A 1662 prescription, Novombergskii, *Materialy,* 1:1–8; 1646 and 1667 import lists, Mamonov, *Materialy,* 3:601–04.

56 González and Vallejo, "The Scorpion in Spanish Folk Medicine."

57 Findlen, *Possessing Nature,* 269.

58 Fabbri, "Treating Medieval Plague," 253.

59 Nappi, "Bolatu's Pharmacy Theriac"; Beckwith, "Tibetan Treacle."

60 Fabbri, "Treating Medieval Plague," 280; Pugliano, "Botanical Artisans." My thanks to Valentina Pugliano for sharing her expertise on theriac with me.

61 Nappi, "Bolatu's Pharmacy Theriac," 763.

62 Fabbri, "Treating Medieval Plague," 252; Rankin, *The Poison Trials,* 23–50.

63 Pugliano, "Pharmacy, Testing," 267–8.

64 Nappi, "Bolatu's Pharmacy Theriac," 753.

65 McVaugh, "Theriac at Montpellier."

66 Broken wind refers to a form of allergic bronchitis that causes wheezing, coughing, and laboured breathing in horses.

67 "одно коренье едят люди от утробы и от мыту, а другое коренье лошадиное – дают лошадям от запалу, а третье коренье зубное – ростет по полям и по огородам." Mamonov, *Materialy,* 3:676–7.

68 Zabivkin, "Travnik."

69 Mamonov, *Materialy*, 2:292–3.

70 Prescriptions of 1660s–1670s, Richter, *Geschichte*, 2:86.

71 Mamonov, *Materialy*, 3:859–60.

72 A 1679 import from Hamburg and Gdansk, Mamonov, *Materialy*, 4:1122–5; 1698 prescription RGADA f. 143, op. 3, ed. khr. 419.

73 Fabbri, "Treating Medieval Plague," 253–4.

74 Records of medicines sent to the Russian army (1736), RGADA f. 346, op. 1, kn. 9, 328-v.

75 Records of medicines sent to the Russian army (1737), RGADA f. 346, op. 1, kn. 4, 257–69; RGADA f. 346, op. 1, kn. 4, 307–08; RGADA f. 346, op. 1, kn. 4, 386–r; RGADA f. 346, op. 1, kn. 4, 388–9v; RGADA f. 346, op. 1, kn. 4, 390–4v; RGADA f. 346, op. 1, kn. 4, 508–9; RGADA f. 346, op. 1, kn. 4, 548–9; RGADA f. 346, op. 1, kn. 7, 495–6; RGADA f. 346, op. 1, kn. 7, 497–9; RGADA f. 346, op. 1, kn. 7, 610–11. 1750 records of medicines sent to the Russian army, RGADA f. 346, op. 1, kn. 9, 209–10; RGADA f. 346, op. 1, kn. 9, 282–3v; RGADA f. 346, op. 1, kn. 132, 437–8v; RGADA f. 346, op. 1, kn. 132, 439–40v; RGADA f. 346, op. 1, kn. 132, 195–7; RGADA f. 346, op. 1, kn. 131, 333–5;

76 GIM Uvar. no. 172, 11r, 13r, 25v.

77 RNB f. 550, O., VI., no. 4.

78 RNB f. 550, Q., VI., no. 12. An alternate translation of the title would be *Reliquary of Medicine.*

79 "No. 76 Teriaca caelestis
На возмущенныхъ излише дхов и гуморов усмирение на утоление болезнь и упокоение неспящихъ недуговъ дается до 1111 [так] гр. [measures added in different hand] в ренском или в каком и оном пристойном пити согласи еще съ No. 25, 72, 82, 88." *Kovchezhets meditsinskii*, RNB f. 550, Q., VI., no. 12. This book has no page numbers, so all references are made to the number of the recipe.

80 RNB f. 550, Q., VI., no. 12. See chapter 2.

81 Stadsarchief Amsterdam, collection no. 6, 97, 98; collection no. 78, 399, 404, 414. See chapter 2.

82 A 1731 comparison of Russian tarif prices of 1724 and 1731, Stadsarchief Amsterdam, collection no. 78, 415.

83 Collis, *The Petrine Instauration*, 268. My thanks to Robert Collis for pointing me towards this sermon.

84 Ibid.

85 Ibid.
86 Zitser, *The Transfigured Kingdom.*
87 See chapter 3.
88 Schiebinger, "Feminist History," 237.
89 Undated inventory, RGADA f. 143, op. 3, ed. khr. 543.
90 RGADA f. 143, op. 2, ed. khr. 1513.
91 RGADA f. 346, op. 1, kn. 9, 67–8; RGADA f. 346, op. 1, kn. 7, 585–v; RGADA f. 346, op. 1, kn. 7, 588–v.
92 RGADA f. 346 op. 1, kn. 4, 411–12.
93 RGADA f. 346 op. 1, kn. 4, 296–9.
94 RGADA f. 346 op. 1, kn. 7, 591.
95 RGADA f. 346 op. 1, kn. 132, 568–70.
96 Dannenfeldt, "Egyptian Mumia," 174.
97 Dannenfeldt, "Egypt and Egyptian Antiquities"; Dannenfeldt, "Egyptian Mumia." On the evolving meanings of the term "mummy" see Heaney, "How to Make an Inca Mummy."
98 The documents mentioning mumia are the following: 1737 RGADA f. 346, op. 1, kn. 4, 296–9. 1737 RGADA f. 346, op. 1, kn. 4, 411–12. 1737 RGADA f. 346, op. 1, kn. 9, 67–8. 1737 RGADA f. 346, op. 1, kn. 7, 585–v. 1737 RGADA f. 346, op. 1, kn. 7, 591. 1737 RGADA f. 346, op. 1, kn. 7, 588–v. 1750 RGADA f. 346, op. 1, kn. 132, 568–70.
99 Levin, "From Corpse to Cult."
100 On Ruysch's anatomical collections, see for example Knoeff, "Touching Anatomy."
101 *PSZ*, 4: 541–2.
102 "таят невежды, чая, что такие уроды родятся от действа диявольскаго, чрез ведовство и порчу: чему быть невозможно, ибо един Творец всея твари Бог, а не диавол, которому ни над каким созданием власти нет; но от повреждения внутренняго, также от страха и мнения матерняго во время бремени, как тому многие есть примеры, чего испужается мать, такие знаки на дитяти бывают," *PSZ*, 5: 541–2.
103 See for example, Finucci, "Performing Modernity."
104 Anemone, "The Monsters of Peter the Great."
105 Ibid., 589–90.

CHAPTER FIVE

1 Hamling and Richardson, *Everyday Objects.*

2 On the materiality of creating books, see for example Scheper, *The Technique of Islamic Bookbinding.* On the material practices of early modern archives, see De Vivo, "Ordering the Archive." On early modern natural history writing as textual objects in relation to natural historical objects, see Pugliano, "Specimen Lists."

3 On East Asian bookbinding see for example Song, "The History and Characteristics"; on Islamic world bookbinding see for example Scheper, *The Technique of Islamic Bookbinding*; on European bookbinding see for example Pickwoad, "Bookbinding."

4 On the formats and different kinds of pre-1700 official Russian documents, see Kozlov et al., *Gosudarstvennost' Rossii*; Shmidt and Kniaz'kov, *Dokumenty deloproizvodstva.*

5 On the creation and formats of manuscript books in premodern Russia, see Stoliarova and Kashtanov, *Kniga v drevnei Rusi.* On book history in early modern Russia more generally, see Luppov, *Kniga v Rossii v XVII veke*; Luppov, *Kniga v Rossii v pervoi chetverti XVIII veka*; Slukhovskii, *Bibliotechnoe delo.*

6 I have previously written about the paperwork practices of the early modern Russian court in Griffin, "Bureaucracy and Knowledge Creation."

7 On literacy in early modern Russia, see Griffin, "In Search of an Audience," 705–07.

8 Kivelson, "What Was *Chernoknizhestvo*?"; Kivelson, *Desperate Magic,* 133–51. The Russian witchcraft trials continued into the eighteenth century. On the eighteenth-century trials, see Smilianskaia, *Volshebniki, bogokhul'niki, eretiki*; Lavrov, *Koldovstvo i religiia.*

9 1664 report on astrology and venesection, RGADA f. 143, op. 2, ed. khr. 738. 1658 autopsy, Mamonov, *Materialy,* 3:694–5. 1643 report on angina, Mamonov, *Materialy,* 1:46. 1664 report on deer horn, RGADA f. 143, op. 2, ed. khr. 734.

10 See for example 1664 report on deer horn. RGADA f. 143, op. 2, ed. khr. 734.

11 Collins's 1665 report on valerian, RGADA f. 143, op. 2, ed. khr. 741; Mamonov, *Materialy,* 3:791–4.

12 A great many works have been written on this topic. On the issue of coffee in Europe, see for example Ellis, *The Coffee House,* 12–24; Spary, *Eat-*

ing the Enlightenment, 51–95. On coffee in Safavid Iran, see Matthee, "Coffee in Safavid Iran." On coffee in the Ottoman Empire, see Mahamid and Nissim, "Sufis and Coffee Consumption."

13 Collins's 1664 report on coffee, RGADA f. 143, op. 2, ed. khr. 734.

14 See for example Collins's 1664 report on obesity. Mamonov, *Materialy*, 3:787–9.

15 Ellis, *The Coffee House*, 134.

16 Collins's 1664 report on coffee, RGADA f. 143, op. 2, ed. khr. 734. On official translating practices in this period, see Watson, *Tradition and Translation*; Maier and Pilger, "Second-Hand Translation for Tsar Aleksej Mixajovich."

17 Matar, *Islam in Britain*, 115–19.

18 Bogdanov, *O krokodilakh v Rossii*, 58; Yoder, "Tea Time In Romanov Russia," 17. My thanks to Audra Yoder for sharing her thesis with me.

19 1665 report on obesity, Mamonov, *Materialy*, 3:787–9.

20 Stolberg, "Abhorreas pinguedinem," 371.

21 Mamonov, *Materialy*, 1:120–3; *AI*, 3:404.

22 1655 Prescription for Prince Iurii Alekseevich Dolgorukii, RGADA f. 143, op. 2, ed. khr. 749. Prescriptions from 1664–65, Mamonov, *Materialy*, 2:278–309. Prescriptions from 1665–66. RGADA f. 143, op. 2, ed. khr. 749.

23 1654 purchase, Mamonov, *Materialy*, 3:631–2; 1655 purchase, Mamonov, *Materialy*, 2:157; Mamonov, *Materialy*, 3:636–9; 1657 purchase, Mamonov, *Materialy*, 3:722–3; 1669 trade, Mamonov, *Materialy*, 3:805–06.

24 Grey, *The Travels of Pietro Della Valle*, 1:4–8. This incident may also be the same one described by the French writer Isaac de la Peirere in 1647. Bruemmer, *The Narwhal*, 117.

25 Sibirtsaev, *Opyt Bibleisko-estestvennoi istorii*, 252–6.

26 For a modern translation of these passages, see for example the *New Revised Standard Version Bible* for the Christian Bible and sefaria.org for the Tanakh. The word "unicorn" is found in early modern English editions of the Christian Bible in the following verses: Numbers 23:22; Deuteronomy 33:17; Psalms 22:21; Psalms 29:6; Psalms 92:10; Isaiah 34:7; Job 39:9–12. Belova, "Edinorog v narodnykh predstavleniiakh,"; Kovtun, Sinitsyna and Fonkich, "Maksim Grek," 105–07.

27 Some modern Christian groups maintain that unicorns are real and are either rare or extinct. See for example https://answersingenesis.org/extinct-animals/unicorns-in-the-bible/ (accessed 15 March 2022).

28 Gotfredsen, *The Unicorn*, 160–01; Shepard, *The Lore of the Unicorn*, 172.

29 On the reclassification of unicorn horns, see Spary, "On the Ironic Specimen."

30 Shepard, *The Lore of the Unicorn*, 34, 121, 139.

31 See for example Pluskowski, "Narwhals or Unicorns?"

32 1655 report on unicorn horn by Graman, RGADA f. 143, op. 2, ed. khr. 147; Mamonov, *Materialy*, 2:157; Mamonov, *Materialy*, 3:636–9. 1658 report of experiment conducted on a unicorn horn, RGADA f. 143, op. 2, ed. khr. 407; RGADA f. 143, op. 2, ed. khr. 306; Mamonov, *Materialy*, 3:696, 722–3; RGADA f. 143, op. 2, ed. khr. 306; Mamonov, *Materialy*, 3:696. Two reports on the unicorn, 1657, RGADA f. 143, op. 2, ed. khr. 194; Mamonov, *Materialy*, 2:160; 1669 report on unicorn horn, RGADA f. 143, op. 2, ed. khr. 850; Mamonov, *Materialy*, 3:805–06.

33 1664 report on the uses of various animal parts in medical drugs, Novombergskii: *Materialy*, 1:54; 1664 report on deer horn. RGADA f. 143, op. 2, ed. khr. 734.

34 Shepard, *The Lore of the Unicorn*, 156.

35 RGADA f. 143, op. 2, ed. khr. 194; Mamonov, *Materialy*, 2:160.

36 Collis, "Magic, Medicine and Authority."

37 Mamonov, *Materialy*, 2:160–2; RGADA f. 143, op. 2, ed. khr. 194.

38 Mamonov, *Materialy*, 2:160–2; RGADA f. 143, op. 2, ed. khr. 194.

39 RGADA f. 143, op. 2, ed. khr. 306; Mamonov, *Materialy*, 3:696.

40 Rankin, *The Poison Trials*; Rankin, "On Anecdote and Antidotes."

41 Shepard, *Lore of the Unicorn*, 118–19, 170.

42 On Aleksei Mikhailovich's legislation, see Oreshnikov, "Danil Gurchin," 50–1; Fil'kin, "Narodnye apteki"; Novombergskii *Ocherki po istorii Aptechnago dela*; Kudakov, "Nekotorye dannye." On the 1685 investigation, see RGADA f. 143, op. 3, ed. khr. 172.

43 On the use of the medical marketplace concept in regard to the early modern world, see for example Jenner, "The Medical Marketplace." Russia used handwritten decrees until 1714. See Franklin, "Printing and Social Control in Russia 2."

44 1628 witchcraft investigation against Andrei Loptunov, Novombergskii: *Materialy*, vol. 3, part 1, 9–12. See chapter 1.

45 1664 witchcraft case against *syn boyarskii* Dmitrii Volodemirov, Novombergskii, *Materialy*, 1:60–1; 1673 collection of witchcraft cases heard by the Investigations Chancery, Mamonov, *Materialy*, 2:494–5; 1699 witchcraft case against peasant Mikhail Grigor'ev, RGADA f. 143, op. 3,

ed. khr. 454; 1703 witchcraft cases against Nataliia Elfimova and Ustinia, RGADA f. 143, op. 2, ed. khr. 1618.

46 1682 investigation into the "heady herb," RGADA f. 143, op. 3, ed. khr. 172; 1699 investigation into the Kitai-gorod markets, RGADA f. 143, op. 3, ed. khr. 462. See chapter 1.

47 On the history of the opening of these private apothecary shops, see Kovrigina, "Apteki i aptekari."

48 Dr Mark Ridley, who worked at the Russian court in the 1590s, states that "zel'ia" can mean a powder, medicine, or spice. See Stone, *A Dictionarie*, 156.

49 "в царствующем граде Москве впредь иным вновь аптекам и Зелейному ряду, что в Китае городе, также и по всем улицам и по перекресткам, лавкам, в которых продавали всякия неупотребныя травы и зелья, будто вместо лекарств, не быть, и те по улицам и по перекресткам лавки все сломать и очистить, а в том Зелейном ряду торговать иными товары, какими пристойно," *PSZ*, iv, 117. Also published in Tkeshelashvili, *Prakticheskoe rukovodstvo*, 22–3.

50 Here Peter the Great is referring to Aleksei Mikhailovich's order establishing the Apothecary Chancery shop and restricting the sale of internal medicines. On this decree, see Fil'kin, "Narodnye apteki"; Novombergskii, *Ocherki po istorii Aptechnago dela*; Kudakov, "Nekotorye dannye."

51 The two branches of the Apothecary Chancery into which the department had been divided in 1673.

52 "в той де его аптеке чинится у него ныне всяким лекарственным вещам от работников его пропажа великая, которые, крадучи, продают в Овошном и в Москотилном и в Зелейном рядах, а по указу де отца Нашего Великаго Государя [т] Алексея Михайловича [т] 181–ого году Февраля 28 числа, каков состоялся в аптекарском приказе в тех вышеписанных рядах в лавках аптекарских лекарств, которыя продаются из старой и из новой аптек, алексиров, водок и масл нутренных держать и продавать не велено, а кто учнет держать и продавать и им явлено быть в жестоком наказанье." Oreshnikov, "Danil Gurchin," 50–1.

53 1679 malpractice case, RGADA f. 143, op. 2, ed. khr. 1251; Oreshnikov, "Danil Gurchin," 47. See chapter 1.

54 "А ныне де в тех рядах торговые люди такие аптекарские ложно протворенные лекарства и всякия масла держать и продают и от той

их продажи лекарств чинится многим людем в неискусстве и повреждение и безвременная трата… не велеть бы в тех вышереченных рядах аптекарских лекарствы и маслы торговать, чтоб всенародному множеству от той их неискусного ведения продажи лекарств проврeждения и безвременныя не было траты." Oreshnikov, "Gurchin," 50–1. This document, along with the licences granted to Albert Tsander in 1713 and I. M. Butvid in 1742, is also published in Tkeshelashvili, *Russkaia farmatsiia.*

55 Mel'gunov, "Iz istorii," 96.

56 The other men granted licences were Gavril Sauls (1702), Mikhail Jessen Arnkil (1704), Aleksei Merkulov (1709), Avraam Rut(s) (1712), Gavriil Byshevskii (1713), and Albert Georg Tsander (1713). See *Opyt istoricheskogo ocherka,* 10–11. On the organization of these early independent pharmacies, see Morozov, "Po povodu organizatsii."

57 *Opyt istoricheskogo ocherka,* 11.

58 Family service in the Apothecary Chancery was relatively common. See Dumschat, *Mediziner,* 249–59; Unkovskaya, *Brief Lives,* 57.

59 Oreshnikov, "Danil Gurchin." See chapter 3.

60 On this history see in particular Bogatyrev, "The Journeys of Ivan Fedorov."

61 Franklin, "Printing and Social Control in Russia 1"; Franklin, "Printing and Social Control in Russia 2"; Franklin, "Printing and Social Control in Russia 3." See also Marker, *Publishing, Printing*; Okenfuss, *The Rise and Fall.*

62 Iliev, "Short History of the Cyrillic Alphabet."

63 1721 decree PSZ, 6:412–13.

64 1721 decree PSZ, 6:412–13; 1729 decree PSZ, 3:219.

65 1729 decree PSZ, 3:219.

66 Griffin, "Every Court an Island?," 314–15. See chapter 3.

67 1648 investigation of Fedor Priadunov RGADA f. 248, op. 7, ed. khr. 423.

68 RGADA f. 248, op. 7, ed. khr. 423. The decree (but not the investigation) is published in PSZ, 3:202–04. On the Mining College, see Graber, "Tsardom of Rock." My thanks to Anna Graber for providing me with a copy of her thesis.

69 RGADA f. 248, op. 7, ed. khr. 423, 418.

70 RGADA f. 248, op. 7, ed. khr. 423.

71 One author who works on medical manuscripts in the seventeenth century and after is A.B. Ippolitova. See for example Ippolitova, *Russkie rukopisnye travniki.* For works on printed medical books, see Grombakh, *Russkaia meditsinskaia literatura*; Renner, *Russische Autokratie.*

72 On the 1708 original see Oreshnikov, "Daniil Gurchin," 54. Copy from the 1720s, BAN Petrine collection. no. 75.

73 "Аптека обозовая или служивая. Собранная вкратце с разныхъ книгъ аптекарских [или лекарскихъ] на ползу служиваго чина людей, и ихъ коней, которою егда лекаря нетъ могутъ сами себе помощи дать во всякихъ своих и конскихъ немощехъ. Издадеся тщаниемъ и трудами, его ц[а]рского величества ц[а]рствующаго града москвы аптекаря Данила Гурчина. В лето от р[о]ж[де]ства хр[и]стова аши году," RNB Pogodin collection, no. 1561, 110.

74 Grombakh, *Russkaia meditsinskaia literatura*, 22–4.

75 Franklin, "Printing and Social Control in Russia 2"; Gusterin, "Pervyi perevodchik"; Griffin, "Alkoran o Magomete."

76 Grombakh, *Russkaia meditsinskaia literatura*, 24.

77 Florinus, *Oeconomus prudens et legalis; Florinova Ekonomiia* (1738). See also the second Russian edition, *Florinova Ekonomiia* (1760).

78 Grombakh, *Russkaia meditsinskaia literatura*, 25; Renner, *Russische Autokratie.*

79 RNB f. 550, Q., VI., no. 12.

80 Griffin, "In Search of an Audience."

81 "каждый человекъ употреблят в не бытий доктора," GIM Zabelin collection, no. 674, 1-v. See also GIM Vakhrameev collection, no. 534; GIM Barsov collection, no. 2238. Griffin, "In Search of an Audience."

82 GIM Zabelin collection, no. 674; Vakhrameev collection, no. 534; GIM Barsov collection, no. 2238.

83 I am grateful to Sarah Bull for her helpful advice on this issue. See for example Jordanova, "Historical Vision in a Digital Age"; Kassell, "Paper Technologies"; Cordell, "'Q i-jtb the Raven'"; Fyfe, "An Archaeology of Victorian Newspapers."

CONCLUSION

1 Mukharji, *Doctoring Traditions.*

2 Koroloff, "In imperio Rutheno."

3 Schiebinger, "Feminist History."

4 See for example Cañizares-Esguerra, "Iberian Science in the Renaissance."

5 Raj, *Relocating Modern Science*; Chakrabarti, *Materials and Medicine.*

6 Chakrabarti, *Materials and Medicine*; Nappi, "Bolatu's Pharmacy"; Gerritsen and Riello, *The Global Lives of Things.*

Bibliography

ARCHIVAL SOURCES

The Netherlands

Stadsarchief Amsterdam [State Archive, Amsterdam]
Collection no. 6, Archief van de Directie van de Moscovische Handel [Archive of the Directorate for trade with Muscovy]
Collection no. 78, Archief van de Directie van de Oostersche Handel en Reederijen [Archive of the Directorate for Eastern Trade and Shipping Companies]

Russia

RGADA Rossiiskii gosudarstvennyi arkhiv drevnikh aktov [Russian State Archive of Ancient Documents, Moscow]
Fond 143 (collection of the Apothecary Chancery)
Fond 346 (collection of the Medical Chancellery)
Fond 188 (Manuscript collection)
Fond 248 (Senate papers)

GIM Gosudarstvennyi istoricheskii muzei [State Historical Museum, Moscow]
E.V. Barsov's manuscript collection
No. 2238 (*Pharmacopoeia,* 18th century)
A.S. Uvarov's manuscript collection
No. 172 (*Domovaia i pokhodnaia apteka,* early 18th century)
I.A. Vakrameev's manuscript collection

No. 534 (*Pharmacopoeia*, 18th century)
I.E. Zabelin's manuscript collection
No. 674 (*Pharmacopoeia*, 18th century)

RGB Rossiiskaia gosudarstvennaia biblioteka [Russian State Library, Moscow]
Fond 37 (T.F. Bol'shakov's collection)
No. 228 (*Pharmacopoeia*, 1700)

RNB Rossiiskaia natsional'naia biblioteka [Russian National Library, St Petersburg]
M.P. Pogodin's collection
No. 1561 (Collection including *Apteka obozovaia ili sluzhivaia*, 18th century)
Fond 550 (Main collection of manuscript books)
Section VI, Octavos, no. 4 (Collection including *Aptechka domovaia*)
Section VI, Octavos, no. 12 (*Kovchezhets meditsinskii*)

BAN Biblioteka Akademii nauk [Library of the Academy of Sciences, St Petersburg]
Petrine Collection
No. 75 (Domovaia i pokhodnaia apteka, 1720s)

Ukraine

TSNB, Tsentral'na naukova biblioteka Kharkivs'kogo natsional'nogo universitetu imeni V.N. Karazina [Central academic library of Kharkiv national university V.N. Karazin, Kharkiv]
Manuscript books
121-p 159/c. http://escriptorium.univer.kharkov.ua/handle/1237075002/1975 (accessed 05/05/2017)

PRINTED SOURCES

Abraham, Lyndy. "The Sources of Arthur Dee's Fasciculus Chemicus (1631)." *Ambix* 41, no. 3 (1994): 135–41.

Abu-Lughod, Janet L. *Before European Hegemony: The World System AD 1250–1350*. New York: Oxford University Press, 1991.

Adelman, Jeremy. "What Is Global History Now?" *Aeon*, 2 March 2017. https://aeon.co/essays/is-global-history-still-possible-or-has-it-had-its-moment (accessed 1 September 2021).

Akasoy, Anna, and Ronit Yoeli-Tlalim. "Along the Musk Routes: Exchanges between Tibet and the Islamic World." *Asian Medicine* 3, no. 2 (2007): 217–40.

Akty istoricheskie, sobrannye i izdannye arkheograficheskuiu kommissieiu. 5 vols. St Petersburg: Tipografiia II-ogo otdeleniia sobsvennoi E.I.V. kantseliarii, 1841–42.

Alexander, John T. "Medical Developments in Petrine Russia." *Canadian–American Slavic Studies* 8, no. 2 (1974): 198–221.

Andaya, Leonard Y. *The World of Maluku: Eastern Indonesia in the Early Modern Period*. Honolulu: University of Hawaii Press, 1993.

Anemone, Anthony. "The Monsters of Peter the Great: The Culture of the St Petersburg Kunstkamera in the Eighteenth Century." *Slavic and East European Journal* 44, no. 4 (2000): 583–602.

Annenkov, N. *Botanicheskii slovar'*. St Petersburg: Tipografiia imperatorskoi Akademii nauk, 1878.

Appleby, John. "Ivan the Terrible to Peter the Great: British Formative Influence on Russia's Medico-Apothecary System." *Medical History* 27 (1983): 289–304.

Arel, Maria Salomon. "Hospitality at the Hands of the Muscovite Tsar: The Welcoming of Foreign Envoys in Early Modern Russia." *Court Historian* 21, no. 1 (2016): 23–43.

Aslanian, Sebouh David. *From the Indian Ocean to the Mediterranean: The Global Trade Networks of Armenian Merchants from New Julfa*. Berkeley: University of California Press, 2014.

Babichenko, Denis. "Kremlevskie tainy: 33-i element." *Itogi*, 17 December 2002, 36–9.

Bäer, Martinus. *Letopis' Moskovskaia*. http://www.vostlit.info/Texts/rus10/Ber/frametext2.htm (accessed 16 June 2021).

Beckwith, Christopher I. "Tibetan Treacle: A Note on Theriac in Tibet." *Tibetan Society Bulletin* 15 (1980): 49–51.

Belova, O.V. "Edinorog v narodnykh predstavleniiakh i knizhnoi traditsii slavian." *Zhivaia starina* 4 (1994): 11–15.

Berry, Lloyd E., and Robert O. Crummey, eds. *Rude and Barbarous Kingdom: Russia in the Accounts of Sixteenth-Century English Voyagers.* Madison: University of Wisconsin Press, 2012.

Bian, He. *Know Your Remedies: Pharmacy and Culture in Early Modern China.* Princeton: Princeton University Press, 2020.

Bishop, W.J. "English Physicians in Russia in the Sixteenth and Seventeenth Centuries." *Proceedings of the Royal Society of Medicine* (1929): 143–52.

Bleichmar, Daniela. "Books, Bodies, and Fields. Sixteenth-Century Transatlantic Encounters with New World *Materia Medica.*" In *Colonial Botany: Science, Commerce, and Politics in the Early Modern World,* ed. Londa Shiebinger and Claudia Swan, 83–99. Philadelphia: University of Pennsylvania Press, 2007.

Bobrova, M.I. "Travniki XVI–XVIII vv. v fonde Tsentral'noi nauchnoi biblioteki Khar'kovskogo gosudarstvennogo universiteta imeni V. N. Karazina." *Metodichnii visnik istorichnogo fakul'tetu Kharkivs'kogo natsional'nogo universitetu im. V.N. Karazina* 9 (2011): 110–17.

Bogatyrev, Sergei. "Ivan IV (1533–1584)." In *The Cambridge History of Russia,* vol. 1: *From Early Rus' to 1689,* ed. Maureen Perrie, 240–63. Cambridge: Cambridge University Press, 2006.

Bogatyrev, Sergei, ed. "Special Issue: The Journeys of Ivan Fedorov: New Perspectives on Early Cyrillic Printing" *Canadian–American Slavic Studies,* 51, no. 2–3 (2017).

Bogdanov, A.B. *Materialy dlia biograficheskogo spravochinka russkikh vrachei XVII–XX vv.* St Petersburg: Izdatel'stvo Evropeiskogo universiteta v Sankt-Peterburge, 2017.

Bogdanov, K.A. *O krokodilakh v Rossii. Ocherki iz istorii zaimstvovanii i ekzotizmov.* Moscow: Novoe literaturnoe obozrenie, 2006.

Bogoiavlenskii, N.A. *Drevnerusskoe vrachevanie v XI–XVIII vv. Istochniki dlia izucheniia istorii russkoi meditsiny.* Moscow: Medgiz, 1960.

Bolkhovitinov, N.N. *Rossiia otkryvaet Ameriky. 1732–1799.* Moscow: Mezhdunarodnye otnosheniia, 1991.

Bolsokhoyeva, N.D. "Medical Faculties of Buryat Buddhist Monasteries." *Ayur Vijnana* 6 (1999): 6–10.

– "Tibetan Medical Schools of the Aga Area (Chita region)." *Asian Medicine* 3, no. 2 (2007): 334–46.

Borschberg, Peter. "The Euro-Asian Trade and Medicinal Usage of Radix Chinaei in the Early Modern Period (ca 1535–1800)." *Review of Culture* 20 (2006): 103–15.

Boterbloem, Kees. *Moderniser of Russia: Andrei Vinius, 1641–1716.* New York: Palgrave Macmillan, 2013.

Boumediene, Samir. *La colonisation du savoir: une histoire des plantes médicinales du 'Nouveau Monde' (1492–1750).* Vaulx-en-Velin: Les éditions des mondes à faire, 2016.

Breen, Benjamin. "Portugal, Early Modern Globalization and the Origins of the Global Drug Trade." *Perspectives on Europe* 42, no. 1 (2012): 84–8.

– "Drugs and Early Modernity." *History Compass* 15, no. 4 (2017): 1–9.

– *The Age of Intoxication: Origins of the Global Drug Trade.* Philadelphia: University of Pennsylvania Press, 2019.

Brostrom, Kenneth N. *Archpriest Avvakum. The Life Written by Himself.* Ann Arbor: Michigan Slavic Publications, 1979.

Brown, Peter B. "Military Planning and High-Level Decision-Making in Seventeenth-Century Russia: The Roles of the Military Chancellery (Razriad) and the Boyar Duma." *Forschungen zur osteuropäischen Geschichte* 58 (2002): 33–43.

Bruemmer, Fred. *The Narwhal. Unicorn of the Sea.* Shrewsbury: Swan Hill Press, 1993.

Bulanin, D.M., and G.M. Prokhorov eds. *Slovar' knizhnikov i knizhnosti drevnei Rusi. Vtoraia polovina XIV–XVI v. chast' 1 A-K.* Moscow: Nauka, 1988.

Burke, Peter. "Cultures of Translation in Early Modern Europe." In *Cultural Translation in Early Modern Europe,* ed. Peter Burke and R. Po-Chia Hsia, 7–38. Cambridge: Cambridge University Press, 2007.

Burton, Audrey. *The Bukharans: A Dynastic, Diplomatic and Commercial History 1550–1702.* Richmond: Curzon Press, 1997.

Cañizares-Esguerra, Jorge. "Iberian Science in the Renaissance: Ignored How Much Longer?" *Perspectives on Science* 12, no. 1 (2004): 86–124.

– ed. *Entangled Empires: The Anglo-Iberian Atlantic, 1500–1830.* Philadelphia: University of Pennsylvania Press, 2018.

Chakrabarti, Pratik. "Empire and Alternatives: Swietenia febrifuga and the Cinchona Substitutes." *Medical History* 54, no. 1 (2010): 75–94.

– *Materials and Medicine: Trade, Conquest and Therapeutics in the Eighteenth Century.* Manchester: Manchester University Press, 2010.

Charters, Erica, Marie Houllemare, and Peter H. Wilson. *A Global History of Early Modern Violence.* Manchester: Manchester University Press, 2020.

Chipman, Leigh. *The World of Pharmacy and Pharmacists in Mamluk Cairo.* Leiden: Brill, 2009.

Chrissidis, Nikolaos A. *An Academy at the Court of the Tsars: Greek Scholars and Jesuit Education in Early Modern Russia*. DeKalb: Northern Illinois University Press, 2015.

Clericuzio, Antonio. "From van Helmont to Boyle. A Study of the Transmission of Helmontian Chemical and Medical Theories in Seventeenth-Century England." *British Journal for the History of Science* 26, no. 3 (1993): 303–34.

Clunas, Craig. *Superfluous Things: Material Culture and Social Status in Early Modern China*. Honolulu: University of Hawaii Press, 2004.

Collins, Daniel E. "Speech Reporting and the Suppression of Orality in Seventeenth- Century Russian Trial Dossiers." *Journal of Historical Pragmatics* 7 (2006): 265–92.

– *Reanimated Voices. Speech Reporting in a Historical-Pragmatic Perspective*. Amsterdam and Philadelphia: John Benjamins, 2001.

Collis, Robert. "Mag elizavetinskoi epokhi: astrologicheskaia kar'era Elizeusa Bomeliusa v 1560-kh godakh." In *Britanskie issledovaniia*. Rostov-on-the-Don: Iuzhnyi federal'nyi universitet, 2010: 154–77.

– *The Petrine Instauration: Religion, Esotericism and Science at the Court of Peter the Great, 1689–1725*. Leiden: Brill, 2011.

– "Magic, Medicine and Authority in Mid-Seventeenth-Century Muscovy: Andreas Engelhardt (d. 1683) and the Role of the Western Physician at the Court of Tsar Aleksei Mikhailovich, 1656–1666." *Russian History* 40 (2013): 399–427.

Cook, Harold J. *Matters of Exchange: Commerce, Medicine, and Science in the Dutch Golden Age*. New Haven: Yale University Press, 2007.

Cook, Harold J., and Timothy D. Walker. "Circulation of Medicine in the Early Modern Atlantic World." *Social History of Medicine* 26, no. 3 (2013): 337–51.

Cooper, Alix. *Inventing the Indigenous: Local Knowledge and Natural History in Early Modern Europe*. Cambridge: Cambridge University Press, 2007.

Cooper, Frederick. "What Is the Concept of Globalization Good For? An African Historian's Perspective." *African Affairs* 100, no. 399 (2001): 189–213.

Cordell, Ryan. "'Q i-jtb the Raven': Taking Dirty OCR Seriously." *Book History* 20, no. 1 (2017): 188–225.

Crawford, Matthew James, and Joseph M. Gabriel. *Drugs on the Page: Pharmacopoeias and Healing Knowledge in the Early Modern Atlantic World*. Pittsburgh: University of Pittsburgh Press, 2019.

Crellin, John K. "Early Settlements in Newfoundland and the Scourge of Scurvy." *Canadian Bulletin of Medical History* 17, no. 1 (2000): 127–36.

Crummey, Robert O. *The Formation of Muscovy 1304–1613*. London and New York: Longman, 1987.

– "The Origins of the Noble Official: The Boyar Elite, 1613–1689." In *Russian Officialdom: The Bureaucratization of Russian Society from the Seventeenth to the Twentieth Century*, ed. Walter McKenzie Pintner and Don Karl Rowney, 46–75. London: MacMillan, 2001.

Culpeper, Nicholas. *Culpeper's Complete Herbal and English Physician*. Carlisle, MA: Applewood Books, 2007.

Dannenfeldt, Karl H. "Egypt and Egyptian Antiquities in the Renaissance." *Studies in the Renaissance* 6 (1959): 7–27.

– "Egyptian Mumia: The Sixteenth Century Experience and Debate." *Sixteenth Century Journal* 16 (1985): 163–80.

Davies, Owen, and Francesca Matteoni. "'A Virtue beyond All Medicine': The Hanged Man's Hand, Gallows Tradition and Healing in Eighteenth- and Nineteenth-Century England." *Social History of Medicine* 28, no. 4 (2015): 686–705.

de Ceglia, Francesco Paolo. "Thinking with the Saint: The Miracle of Saint Januarius of Naples and Science in Early Modern Europe." *Early Science and Medicine* 19, no. 2 (2014): 133–73.

De Laet, Marianne, and Annemarie Mol. "The Zimbabwe Bush Pump: Mechanics of a Fluid Technology." *Social Studies of Science* 30, no. 2 (2000): 225–63.

de Madariaga, Isabel. *Ivan the Terrible: First Tsar of Russia*. London: Yale University Press, 2006.

Demidova, N.F. "Buriokratizatsiia gosudarstvennogo apparata absoliutizma v XVII–XVIII vv." In *Absoliutizm v Rossii XVII–XVIII vv: Sbornik statei k semidesiatiletiiu so dnia rozhdeniia i sorokapiatiletiiu nauchnoi i pedagogicheskoi deiatel'nosti B.B. Kafengauza*, ed N. M. Druzhinin, 206–42. Moscow: Nauka, 1964.

– *Sluzhilaia biurokratiia v Rossii XVII v. i ee rol' v formirovanii abosoliutizma*. Moscow: Nauka, 1987.

De Vivo, Filippo. "Ordering the Archive in Early Modern Venice (1400–1650)." *Archival Science* 10, no. 3 (2010): 231–48.

De Vos, Paula. "From Herbs to Alchemy: The Introduction of Chemical Medicine to Mexican Pharmacies in the Seventeenth and Eighteenth Centuries." *Journal of Spanish Cultural Studies* 8, no. 2 (2007): 135–68.

De Vries, Jan. "The Limits of Globalization in the Early Modern World." *Economic History Review* 63, no. 3 (2010): 710–33.

De Zwart, Pim, and Jan Luiten van Zanden. *The Origins of Globalization: World Trade in the Making of the Global Economy, 1500–1800*. Cambridge: Cambridge University Press, 2018.

Debus, Allen G. *The Chemical Philosophy: Paracelsian Science and Medicine in the Sixteenth and Seventeenth Centuries.* Mineola: Dover Publications, 1977.

– *The French Paracelsians: The Chemical Challenge to Medical and Scientific Tradition in Early Modern France.* Cambridge: Cambridge University Press, 2002.

Dee, Arthur, *Fasciculus chemicus, abstrusae Hermeticae scientiae, ingressum, progressum, coronidem verbis apertissimis explicans, etc.* Stetini: typis [et] impensis Dauidis Rehtii, 1644.

Dmitrieva, R.P., ed. *Povest' o Petre i Fevronii: Podgotovka tekstov i issledovanie* Leningrad: Nauka, 1979.

Dooley, Brendan. "Social Control and the Italian Universities: From Renaissance to Illuminismo." *Journal of Modern History* 61 (1989): 205–39.

Dörbeck, Franz, "Origin of Medicine in Russia." *Medical Life* 30 (1923): 223–34.

Dorwart, Reinhold A. "The Royal College of Medicine and Public Health in Brandenburg-Prussia, 1685–1740." *Medical History* 2, no. 1 (1958): 13–23.

Drayton, Richard, and David Motadel. "Discussion: The Futures of Global History." *Journal of Global History* 13, no. 1 (2018): 1–21.

Dubcovsky, Alejandra, and George Aaron Broadwell. "Writing Timucua: Recovering and Interrogating Indigenous Authorship." *Early American Studies: An Interdisciplinary Journal* 15, no. 3 (2017): 409–41.

Dumschat, Sabine. *Ausländischer Mediziner im Moskauer Russland.* Stuttgart: Franz Steiner Verlag, 2006.

Dunning, Chester S.L. *Russia's First Civil War: The Time of Troubles and the Founding of the Romanov Dynasty*. University Park: Pennsylvania State Press, 2010.

– trans. and ed. *Jacques Margeret, The Russian Empire and Grand Duchy of Muscovy. A 17th-Century French Account.* Pittsburgh: University of Pittsburgh Press, 1983.

Earle, Rebecca. *The Body of the Conquistador: Food, Race and the Colonial Experience in Spanish America, 1492–1700*. Cambridge: Cambridge University Press, 2012.

Edwards, John I. "Looking for Abram Hannibal: Some Observations on the Supposed Portraits of Abram Petrovich Hannibal (1696–1781) the

African Great-Grandfather of Aleksandr Pushkin." *Slavonica* 9, no. 1 (2003): 19–33.

Ellis, Markman. *The Coffee House: A Cultural History*. London: Weidenfeld & Nicolson, 2011.

Emchenko, E.B., *Stoglav: Issledovanie i tekst*. Moscow: Indrik, 2000.

Eugène-Humbert, Guitard. "Les serments professionnels de la pharmacie de l'antiquité à nos jours (suite et fin)." *Revue d'histoire de la pharmacie*, 35e année, no. 117 (1947): 122–32.

Fabbri, Christiane Nockels. "Treating Medieval Plague: The Wonderful Virtues of Theriac." *Early Science and Medicine* 12, no. 3 (2007): 247–83.

Fan, F.T. "The Global Turn in the History of Science." *East Asian Science, Technology and Society: An International Journal* 6, no. 2 (2012): 249–58.

Fauvelle, François-Xavier. *The Golden Rhinoceros: Histories of the African Middle Ages*. Princeton: Princeton University Press, 2018.

Figurovskii, Nikolai Aleksandrovich. "The Alchemist and Physician Arthur Dee (Artemii Ivanovich Dii): An Episode in the History of Chemistry and Medicine in Russia." *Ambix* 13, no. 1 (1965): 35–51.

– "The History of Chemistry in Ancient Russia." *Chymia* 11 (1966): 45–79.

Fil'kin, A.M., "Narodnye apteki Moskovskogo gosudarstva XVII veka." *Farmatsiia* 18 (1969): 52–5.

Findlen, Paula. *Possessing Nature: Museums, Collecting, and Scientific Culture in Early Modern Italy*. Berkeley, Los Angeles and London: University of California Press, 1994.

Finucci, Valeria. *The Manly Masquerade: Masculinity, Paternity, and Castration in the Italian Renaissance*. London: Duke University Press, 2003.

Fissell, Mary E. "The Marketplace of Print." In *Medicine and the Market in England and Its Colonies, c.1450–c.1850*, ed Mark Jenner and Patrick Wallis, 108–32. Basingstoke: Palgrave Macmillan, 2007.

Florinova Ekonomiia, s nemetskago na rossiiskoi iazyk sokrashcheno perevedena i napechatana poveleniem eia Imperatorskago Velichestva Vsemilotsiveishiia Velikiia Gosudaryni Imperatritsy Anny Ioannovny Samoderzhitsy Vserossiiskia. St Petersburg: Imperatorskaia Akademiia Nauk, 1738.

Florinova Ekonomiia v deviati knigakh sostoiashchaia; s nemetskago na rossiiskoi iazyk sokrashcheno Sergiem Volchkovym. Izdanie vtoroe. St Petersburg: Imperatorskaia Akademiia Nauk, 1760.

Florinskii, V.M. *Russkie prostonarodnye travniki i lechebniki. Sobranie meditsinskikh rukopisei XVI i XVII stoletiia*. Kazan: Tipografiia Imperatorskogo universiteta, 1879.

Florinus, Franz Philipp, *Oeconomus prudens et legalis. Oder Allgemeiner Klug-*

und Rechts-verständiger Haus-Vatter: bestehend In Neun Büchern. Frankfurt: Riegel, 1702.

Flynn, Dennis O., and Arturo Giráldez. "Globalization Began in 1571." *Globalization and Global History* (2006): 232–47.

Fors, Hjalmar. "Medicine and the Making of a City: Spaces of Pharmacy and Scholarly Medicine in Seventeenth-Century Stockholm." *Isis* 107, no. 3 (2016): 473–94.

Foust, Clifford M. *Rhubarb: The Wondrous Drug.* Princeton: Princeton University Press, 1992.

Franklin, Simon. "Printing and Social Control in Russia 1: Passports." *Russian History* 37, no. 3 (2010): 208–37.

– "Printing and Social Control in Russia 2: Decrees." *Russian History* 38, no. 4 (2011): 467–92.

– "Printing Social Control in Russia 3: Blank Forms." *Russian History* 42, no. 1 (2015): 114–35.

French, Peter. *John Dee: The World of the Elizabethan Magus.* London and New York: Routledge, 2013.

Frost, Kate. "Prescription and Devotion: The Reverend Doctor Donne and the Learned Doctor Mayerne – Two Seventeenth-Century Records of Epidemic Typhus Fever." *Medical History* 22, no. 4 (1978): 408–16.

Fyfe, Paul. "An Archaeology of Victorian Newspapers." *Victorian Periodicals Review* 49, no. 4 (2016): 546–77.

Gänger, Stefanie. "World Trade in Medicinal Plants from Spanish America, 1717–1815." *Medical History* 59, no. 1 (2015): 44–62.

Geary, Patrick. "Sacred Commodities: The Circulation of Medieval Relics." In *The Social Life of Things: Commodities in Cultural Perspective,* ed. Arjun Appadurai, 169–91. Cambridge: Cambridge University Press, 1986.

Gerasimov, M.M. "Dokumental'nyi portret Ivana Groznogo." *Kratkie soobshcheniia Instituta arkheologii AN SSSR* 100 (1965): 139–42.

– "Portrety istoricheskikh lits." *Nauka i chelovechestvo* (1965): 97–119.

Gerritsen, Anne, and Giorgio Riello. *The Global Lives of Things: The Material Culture of Connections in the Early Modern World.* London: Routledge, 2015.

Gnammankou, Dieudonné. *Abraham Hanibal: l'aïeul noir de Pouchkine.* Paris: Présence Africaine, 1996.

Goldstein, Darra. "Gastronomic Reforms under Peter the Great. Toward a Cultural History of Russian Food." *Jahrbücher für Geschichte Osteuropas* H. 4 (2000): 481–510.

González, José A., and José Ramón Vallejo. "The Scorpion in Spanish Folk

Medicine: A Review of Traditional Remedies for Stings and Its Use as a Therapeutic Resource." *Journal of Ethnopharmacology* 146, no. 1 (2013): 62–74.

Gordin, Michael D. "The Importation of Being Earnest: The Early St Petersburg Academy of Sciences." *Isis* 91, no. 1 (2000): 1–31.

Gotfredsen, Lise. *The Unicorn*. Trans. Anne Born. London: Harvill Press, 1999.

Graber, Anna, "Tsardom of Rock: State, Society, and Mineral Science in Enlightenment Russia." Unpublished PhD diss., Yale University, 2016.

Graber, Anna, Clare Griffin, Rachel Koroloff, and Audra Yoder. "Introduction: The Natural Turn in Early Modern Russian History." *ВИВЛІОѲИКА: E-Journal of Eighteenth-Century Russian Studies* 6 (2018): 1–12.

Graham, Loren R. *Science in Russia and the Soviet Union: A Short History*. Cambridge: Cambridge University Press, 1993.

Granel H. "Un serment d'apothicaire en 1645." *Bulletin de la Société d'histoire de la pharmacie* 7e année, no. 23 (1919): 1.

Green, Monica H. "Editor's Introduction to Pandemic Disease in the Medieval World: Rethinking the Black Death." *Medieval Globe* 1, no. 1 (2014): 9–26.

– "Taking 'Pandemic' Seriously: Making the Black Death Global." *Medieval Globe* 1, no. 1 (2014): 27–62.

Grek, Maxim. *Sochinenia*. Kazan, 1862.

Grell, Ole Peter, Andrew Cunningham, and Jon Arrizabalaga, eds. *It All Depends on the Dose: Poisons and Medicines in European History*. New York: Routledge, 2018.

Grey, Edward, ed. *The Travels of Pietro Della Valle in India. From the Old English Translation of 1664*. Cambridge: Cambridge University Press, 2010.

Griffin, Clare. "The Production and Consumption of Medical Knowledge in Seventeenth-Century Russia: The Apothecary Chancery." Unpublished PhD diss., University College London, 2013.

– "In Search of an Audience: Popular Pharmacies and the Limits of Literate Medicine in Late Seventeenth- and Early Eighteenth-Century Russia." *Bulletin of the History of Medicine* 89, no. 4 (2015): 705–32.

– "Povest' preslavna, 'The wondrous tale.'" *Christian–Muslim Relations: A Bibliographical History*, vol. 8: *Northern and Eastern Europe (1600–1700)*, ed. David Thomas and John Chesworth, 841–2. Leiden: Brill, 2016.

– "Bureaucracy and Knowledge Creation: The Apothecary Chancery." In *Information and Empire: Mechanisms of Communication in Russia, 1600–1850*, ed. Simon Franklin and Katherine Bowers, 255–85. Cambridge: Open Book Publishers, 2017.

– "Every Court an Island? Palace Medicine, International Exchanges, and Popular Practices in Early Modern Russia." *Medizinhistorisches Journal* 53, no. 3–4 (2018): 309–30.

– "Russia and the Medical Drug Trade in the Seventeenth Century." *Social History of Medicine* 31, no. 1 (2018): 2–23.

– "Such a Pretty Tsaritsa," *Nursing Clio*. 2020. https://nursingclio.org/2020/07/01/such-a-pretty-tsaritsa/.

– "'Pyotr Vasilevich Postnikov' and 'The Al-Koran on Muhammad,'" *Christian–Muslim Relations: A Bibliographical History*, vol. 8: *Northern and Eastern Europe (1600–1700)*, ed. David Thomas and John Chesworth, 605–7. Leiden: Brill, 2020.

– "Disentangling Commodity Histories: Pauame and Sassafras in the Early Modern Global World." *Journal of Global History* 15, no. 1 (2020): 1–18.

– "The Unexotic World: Medical Drugs, Global Exchanges, and Moscow's View of the Foreign, c. 1690." In *Exoticizing Consumption: European Drug Cultures around 1700*, ed. Emma Spary and Justin Rivest, forthcoming.

Grombakh, S.M. *Russkaia meditsinskaia literatura XVIII veka*. Moscow: Akademia meditsinskikh nauk, 1953.

Gruzdev, V.F., *Russkie rukopisnye travniki*. Leningrad: Voenno-morskoi meditsinskaia akademiia, 1946.

Gusterin, P.V. "Pervyi perevodchik i pervoe izdanie Korana na russkom iazyke." *Islamovedenie* 1 (2011): 89–97.

Haigh, Basil. "Design for a Medical Service: Peter the Great's Admiralty Regulations (1722)." *Medical History* 19, no. 2 (1975): 129–46.

Hamling, Tara, and Catherine Richardson, eds. *Everyday Objects: Medieval and Early Modern Material Culture and Its Meanings*. Farnham: Ashgate, 2010.

Heaney, Christopher. "How to Make an Inca Mummy: Andean Embalming, Peruvian Science, and the Collection of Empire." *Isis* 109, no. 1 (2018): 1–27.

Hedesan, Georgiana D. "Alchemy, Potency, Imagination: Paracelsus's Theories of Poison." In *It All Depends on the Dose: Poisons and Medicines in European History*, ed. Ole Peter Grell, Andrew Cunningham, and Jon Arrizabalaga, 81–102. New York: Routledge, 2018.

Hellie, Richard, "In Search of Ivan the Terrible." In *Ivan the Terrible*, ed. S.F. Platonov, ix–xxxiv. Gulf Breeze, FL: Academic International Press, 1974.

– *The Economy and Material Culture of Russia, 1600–1725*. Chicago: University of Chicago Press, 1999.

Heng, Geraldine. "Early Globalities, and Its Questions, Objectives, and Methods: An Inquiry into the State of Theory and Critique." *Exemplaria* 26, no. 2–3 (2014): 234–53.

Herzberg, Julia. "Faith on the Menu: Conflicts around Fasting in Muscovy." *Kritika: Explorations in Russian and Eurasian History* 21, no. 2 (2020): 371–400.

Hortius, Johannes Daniel. *Pharmacopoiea Galeno-Chemica post Renodaeum Quertanum aliosque huius generis celeberrimos utriusque medicinae doctores practicos adornata selectissimisque medicamentorum compositionibus, experimentis, et observationibus Spagyricis rarissimis et novis, nec non morborum omnium appropriatis remedis probatissimis adaucta. Accesserunt institutiones pharmaceuticae Methodo elegantissima praeparandi.* Frankfurt, 1651.

Hughes, Lindsey. *Russia in the Age of Peter the Great.* New Haven: Yale University Press, 1998.

Huguet-Termes, Teresa. "New World Materia Medica in Spanish Renaissance Medicine: From Scholarly Reception to Practical Impact." *Medical History* 45, no. 3 (2001): 359–76.

Hulkower, Raphael. "The History of the Hippocratic Oath: Outdated, Inauthentic, and Yet Still Relevant." *Einstein Journal of Biology and Medicine* 25, no. 1 (2010): 41–4.

Iliev, Ivan G. "Short History of the Cyrillic Alphabet." *International Journal of Russian Studies* 2, no. 2 (2013): 1–65.

Iosad, Alexander. "'Sciences Strange and Diverse': Europeanization through the Transfer of Scientific Knowledge in Russia, 1717–65." Unpublished PhD diss., University of Oxford, 2017.

Ippolitova, A.B., *Russkie rukopisnye travniki XVII–XVIII vekov. Issledovanie fol'klora i etnobotaniki.* Moscow: Indrik, 2008.

Isachenko, T.A. *Prokhladnyi vertograd. Lechebnik patriarshego keleinika Filagriia.* Moscow: Arkheograficheskii tsentr, 1997.

– "Travnik Nikolaia Liubchanina i ego sud'ba na russkoi pochve." *Drevniaia Rus'. Voprosy medievistiki* 36 (2009): 97–109.

– *Perevodnaia Moskovskaia knizhnost'. Mitropolichii i patriarshii skriptorii XV–XVII vv.* Moscow: Rossiiskaia gosudarstvennaia biblioteka, 2009.

– "Ruskopisi mitropolich'ego skriptoriia v bibliotekakh Rossii i Litvy (k istorii unikal'noi vil'niusskoi rukopisi tsarskogo travnika)." *Knygotyra* (2010): 186–98.

Jenner, Mark S.R., and Patrick Wallis. "The Medical Marketplace." In *Medicine and the Market in England and Its Colonies, c. 1450–c. 1850*, ed. Mark S.R. Jenner and Patrick Wallis, 1–23. London: Palgrave Macmillan, 2007.

Johnston Pouncy, Carolyn, ed. and trans. *The Domostroi: Rules for Russian Households in the Time of Ivan the Terrible.* Ithaca: Cornell University Press, 1994.

Jordanova, Ludmilla. "Historical Vision in a Digital Age." *Cultural and Social History* 11, no. 3 (2014): 343–8.

Kaiser, Daniel H. *Death and Dying in Early Modern Russia*. Washington, DC: Wilson Center, Kennan Institute, 1987.

Karoly, László. *A Turkic Medical Treatise from Islamic Central Asia: A Critical Edition of a Seventeenth-Century Chagatay Work by Subḥān Qulï Khan*. Leiden: Brill, 2014.

Karpenko, Vladimor, and John A. Norris. "Vitriol in the History of Chemistry." *Chemické listy* 96, no. 12 (2002): 997–1005.

Kassell, Lauren. "Paper Technologies, Digital Technologies: Working with Early Modern Medical Records." In *The Edinburgh Companion to the Critical Medical Humanities*, ed. Anne Whitehead, Angela Woods, Jennifer Richards, Sarah Atkinson, and Jane Macnaughton, 120–35. Edinburgh University Press, 2016.

Keenan, Edward L. "Vita. Ivan Vasilevich, Terrible Tsar: 1530–1584." *Harvard Magazine* 80, no.3 (1978): 48–9.

Keenan, Edward. "Ivan IV and the 'King's Evil': Ni Maka Li To Budet?" *Russian History* 20, no. 1–4 (1993): 5–13.

Keenan, Edward L., and Russell E. Martin. "The Tsar's Two Bodies." *Canadian-American Slavic Studies* 51, no. 1 (2017): 3–28.

Keränen, Lisa. "The Hippocratic Oath as Epideictic Rhetoric: Reanimating Medicine's Past for Its Future." *Journal of Medical Humanities* 22, no. 1 (2001): 55–68.

Khoteev, P.I. "Biblioteka Leib-medika I.G. Lestoka." In *Kniga i biblioteki v Rossii v XIV – pervoi polovine XIX v.*, ed. S.P. Luppov et al., 42–55. Leningrad: Biblioteka Akademii nauk, 1982.

Khudin, K.S. "Stanovleniie mozhzhevelovoi povinnosti v Rossii v XVII v. (po materialam fonda Aptekarskogo prikaza RGADA)." *Vestnik RGGU. Seriia "Istoriia. Filologiia. Kulturologiia"* 21 (2012): 118–26.

– "Dokumenty aptekarskogo prikaza v sobranii arkhiva Sankt-Petersburgskogo Instituta Istorii (SpbII) RAN (1654–1655 gg.): po materialam "Kollektsii moskovskikh aktov" (k. 249) i "kollektsii N.P. Likhacheva" (k. 238)." *Vestnik RGGU. Seriia "Istoriia. Filologiia. Kulturologiia"* no. 9 (2015): 90–6.

– "Retsepty Aptekarskogo prikaza XVII v. kak istoricheskii istochnik: istochnikovedcheskii potentsial." in *Istoriia Rossii s drevneishikh vremen do XXI veka: problem, diskusii, novye vzgliady*, ed. Yu.A. Petrov and V.N. Kruglov, 44–9. Moscow: Institut rossiiskoi istorii RAN, 2018.

– "Lechenie kornem "Zaiach'e kopyto" Boriarina B.I. Morozova (1661 g.)." *Acta Linguistica Petropolitana* 13, no. 2 (2017): 387–94.

– "Nomenklatura lekarstvennykh rastenii v meditsinskoi praktike Aptekarskogo prikaza (na materiale retseptov dlia datskogo korolevicha Vol'demara 1644–1645 gg.)." *Acta Linguistica Petropolitana* 13, no. 2 (2017): 396–415.
– "Nazvaniia lekarstvennykh rastenii v istochnikakh o Russko-indiiskoi torgovle XVII v. (po dokumentam Aptekarskogo prikaza)." *Acta Linguistica Petropolitana* 15, no. 3 (2019): 461–88.
Kivelson, Valerie A. "Political Sorcery in Sixteenth-Century Muscovy." In *Culture and Identity in Muscovy, 1359–1584*, ed. A.M. Kleimola and G.D. Lenhoff, 267–83. Moscow: ITZ-Garant, 1997.
– *Cartographies of Tsardom: The Land and Its Meanings in Seventeenth-Century Russia*. Ithaca: Cornell University Press, 2006.
– "'Between All Parts of the Universe': Russian Cosmographies and Imperial Strategies in Early Modern Siberia and Ukraine." *Imago Mundi* 60, no. 2 (2008): 166–81.
– "What Was *Chernoknizhestvo*? Black Books and Foreign Writings in Muscovite Magic." In *Rude and Barbarous Kingdom Revisited*, ed. Chester Dunning, Russell Martin, and Daniel Rowland, 1–15. Bloomington: Slavica, 2008.
– *Desperate Magic: The Moral Economy of Witchcraft in Seventeenth-Century Russia*. Ithaca: Cornell University Press, 2013.
Kleimola, Ann M. "The Duty to Denounce in Muscovite Russia." *Slavic Review* 31, no. 4 (1972): 759–79.
Knoeff, Rina. "Touching Anatomy: On the Handling of Preparations in the Anatomical Cabinets of Frederik Ruysch (1638–1731)." *Studies in History and Philosophy of Science Part C: Studies in History and Philosophy of Biological and Biomedical Sciences* 49 (2015): 32–44.
Knöpfler, J.Frz. "Eidesformeln für Arzt, Apotheker, Hebammen, Wundarzt und Frauenwirt zu Amberg aus dem 15. Jahrh. – Taxordnung für den Stadtarzt daselbst, 1561; Sondersiechenordnung von Amberg vom Jahre 1582." *Archiv für Geschichte der Medizin* Bd. 11, H. 5/6, September 1919: 318–24.
Kobrin, V.B. *Ivan Groznyi*. Moscow: Moskovskie rabochie, 1989.
Kolesov, V.V., and V.V. Rozhdestvenskaia. *Domostroi*. St Petersburg: Nauka, 1994.
Kolosova, V.B. "Name-Text-Ritual: The Role of Plant Characteristics in Slavic Folk Medicine." *Folklorica* 10, no. 2 (2005): 44–61.
Koroloff, Rachel. *Seeds of Exchange: Collecting for Russia's Apothecary and Botanical Gardens in the Seventeenth and Eighteenth Centuries*. Unpublished PhD diss., University of Illinois at Urbana-Champaign, 2015.

– "'In imperio Rutheno': Johann Amman's *Stirpium rariorum* (1739) and the Foundation of Russia's Botanical Empire." In *The Botany of Empire in the Long Eighteenth Century*, ed. Yota Batsaki, Sarah Burke Cahalan, and Anatole Tchikine, 235–56. Washington, DC: Dumbarton Oaks Research Library and Collection, 2017.

– "The Patriarchy and the Apothecary: Planting Gardens and Making Holy Miro in Seventeenth-Century Moscow." In *Sound and Scent in the Garden*, ed. D. Fairchild Ruggles, 153–70. Washington, DC: Dumbarton Oaks Research Library and Collection, 2017.

– "Travniki, Travniki and Travniki: Herbals, Herbalists and Herbaria in Seventeenth-Century and Eighteenth-Century Russia." *ВИВЛІОθИКА: E-Journal of Eighteenth-Century Russian Studies* 6 (2018): 58–76.

– "Juniper: From Medicine to Poison and Back Again in 17th-Century Muscovy." *Kritika: Explorations in Russian and Eurasian History* 19, no. 4 (2018): 697–716.

Kotilaine, Jarmo T. *Russia's Foreign Trade and Economic Expansion in the Seventeenth Century: Windows on the World.* Leiden: Brill, 2005.

Kotkova, S.I. *Vesti-Kuranty, 1645–46, 1648g.* Moscow: Nauka, 1980.

Kovrigina, V.A. "Apteki i aptekari Moskvy vtoroi poloviny XVII – pervoi chetverti XVIII v." *Vestnik Moskovskogo universiteta seriia 8 Istoriia* 1 (1999): 38–70.

Kovtun, L.S., N.S. Sinitsyna, and V.L. Fonkich. "Maksim Grek i slavianskaia Psaltyr (Slozhenie norm literaturnogo iazyka v perevodcheskoi praktike XVI v.)." In *Vostochnoslavianskie iazyki. Istochniki dlia ikh izucheniia*, ed. L.P. Zhukovskaia and N.I. Tarabasova, 105–7. Moscow: Nauka, 1973.

Kozlov, O.F. et al., *Gosudarstvennost' Rossii: gosudarstvennye i tserkovnye uchrezhdeniia, soslovnye organy i organy mestnogo samoupravleniia, edinitsy administrativno-territorial'nogo, tserkovnogo i vedomstvennogo deleniia (konets XV veka – fevral' 1917 goda): slovar'-spravochnik.* 6 vols. Moscow: Nauka, 1996–2009.

Küçük, B. Harun. "Eleven. New Medicine and the Ḥikmet-i Ṭabīʿiyye Problematic in Eighteenth-Century Istanbul." In *Texts in Transit in the Medieval Mediterranean*, ed. Y. Tzvi Langermann and Robert G. Morrison, 222–42. University Park, PA: Penn State University Press, 2021.

Kudakov, N.A., "Nekotorye dannye o voznikovenii kontrolia kachestva lekarstvennykh veshchestv na Rusi." *Aptechnoe delo* 5 (1953): 53–5.

Lokhteva, G.N. "Materialy Aptekarskogo prikaza." In *Estestvennonauchnye znaniia v drevnei Rusi*, ed. R.A. Simonov. Moscow: Nauka, 1980.

Lavrov, A.S. *Koldovstvo i religiia v Rossii, 1700–1740 gg.* Moscow: Drevlekhranilishhe, 2000.

Leeming, Henry. "Polish and Polish-Latin Medical Terms in Pre-Petrine Russian." *Slavonic and East European Review* 42 (1963): 89–109.

Lenhoff, Gail. "The Notion of 'Uncorrupted Relics' in Early Russian Culture." In *Christianity and the Eastern Slavs*, vol. 1, ed. Boris Gasparov and Olga Raevsky-Hughes, 252–66. Berkeley: University of California Press, 1993.

Levi, Scott Cameron. *The Indian Diaspora in Central Asia and Its Trade, 1550–1900*. Leiden: Brill, 2002.

Levin, Eve. "Supplicatory Prayers as a Source for Popular Religious Culture in Muscovite Russia." In *Religion and Culture in Early Modern Russia and Ukraine*, ed. Samuel H. Baron and Nancy Shields Kollmann, 96–114. DeKalb: Northern Illinois University Press, 1997.

– "From Corpse to Cult in Early Modern Russia." In *Orthodox Russia: Belief and Practice under the Tsars*, ed. Valerie A. Kivelson and Robert H. Greene, 81–104. University Park: Pennsylvania State University Press, 2003.

– "The Administration of Western Medicine in Seventeenth-Century Russia." In *Modernizing Muscovy. Reform and Social Change in Seventeenth Century Russia*, ed. Jarmo Kotilaine and Marshall Poe, 363–89. London and New York: Routledge Curzon, 2004.

– "Innocent and Demon-Possessed in Early Modern Russia." In *Culture and Identity in Eastern Christian History: Papers from the First Biennial Conference of the Association for the Study of Eastern Christian History and Culture (ASEC), Inc.*, ed. Russell E. Martin and Jennifer Spock, with the assistance of M.A. Johnson, 123–62. Columbus: Department of Slavic and East European Languages and Literatures, OSU, 2009.

– "Healers and Witches in Early Modern Russia." In *Saluting Aron Gurevich: Essays in History, Literature, and Other Related Subjects*, ed. Yelena Mazour-Matusevich and Alexandra S. Korros, 105–33. Leiden: Brill, 2010.

Liseitsev, D.V. *Posol'skii prikaz v epokhu smuty*. Moscow: RAN, 2003.

– "Evoliutsiia prikaznoi sistemy Moskovskogo gosudarstva v epokhu Smuty." *Otechestvennaia istoriia* 1 (2006): 3–15.

Liseitsev, D.V., N.M. Rogozhin, and Iu.M. Eskin. *Prikazy Moskovskogo gosudarstva XVI–XVII vv. Slovar'-spravochnik*. Moscow and St Petersburg: Tsentr gumanitarnykh initsiativ, 2015.

Liubimenko, Inna. "Vrachebnoe i lekarstvennoe delo v Moskovskom gosudarstve." *Russkii istoricheskii zhurnal* 1 (1917): 3–36.

Luppov, S.P., *Kniga v Rossii v XVII veke* Leningrad: Nauka, 1970.

– *Kniga v Rossii v pervoi chetverti XVIII veka* Leningrad: Nauka, 1973.

Maehle, Andreas-Holger. *Drugs on Trial: Experimental Pharmacology and Therapeutic Innovation in the Eighteenth Century*. Atlanta/Amsterdam: Editions Rodopi B.V., 1999.

Mahamid, Hatim, and Chaim Nissim. "Sufis and Coffee Consumption: Religio-Legal and Historical Aspects of a Controversy in the Late Mamluk and Early Ottoman Periods." *Journal of Sufi Studies* 7, no. 1–2 (2018): 140–64.

Maier, Ingrid. "Newspaper Translations in Seventeenth-Century Muscovy. About the Sources, Topics and Periodicity of *Kuranty* 'Made in Stockholm' (1649)." In *Explorare necesse est. Hyllningsskrift till Barbro Nilsson (Stockholm Slavic Studies XXVIII)*, ed. Per Ambrosiani, Elisabeth Löfstrand, Laila Nordquist, and Ewa Teodorowicz-Hellman, 181–190. Stockholm: Acta Universitatis Stockholmiensis, 2002.

Maier, Ingrid, and Wouter Pilger, "Second-Hand Translation for Tsar Aleksej Mixajlovich – a Glimpse into the 'Newspaper Workshop' at Posol'skij Prikaz." *Russian Linguistics* 25 (2001): 209–42.

Maier, Ingrid, and Daniel C. Waugh. "How Well Was Muscovy Connected with the World?" In *Imperienvergleich. Beispiele und Ansätze aus osteuropäischer Perspektive. Festschrift für Andreas Kappeler*, ed. G. Hausmann and A. Rustemeyer, 17–38. Wiesbaden: Forschungen zur osteuropäischen Geschichte, Band 75, 2009.

Maier, Ingrid, et al. *Vesti-Kuranty, 1656 g., 1660–1662 gg., 1664–1670 gg.* 2 vols. Moscow: Iazyki slavianskikh kul'tur, 2008–9.

Mamonov, N.E. *Materialy dlia istorii medistiny v Rossii*. 4 vols. St Petersburg: M.M. Stasiulevich, 1881.

Margeret, Jacques. *Estat de l'empire de Rvssie, et grande dvche de Moscovie*. Paris, 1669.

Marker, Gary. *Publishing, Printing, and the Origins of the Intellectual Life in Russia, 1700–1800*. Princeton: Princeton University Press, 1985.

Martin, Janet. *Treasure of the Land of Darkness: The Fur Trade and Its Significance for Medieval Russia*. Cambridge: Cambridge University Press, 2004.

Matar, Nabil. *Islam in Britain, 1558–1685*. Cambridge: Cambridge University Press, 1998.

Matthee, Rudi. "Coffee in Safavid Iran: Commerce and Consumption." *Journal of the Economic and Social History of the Orient* 37, no. 1 (1994): 1–32.

McVaugh, Michael. "Theriac at Montpellier 1285–1325 (with an edition of the 'Questiones de tyriaca' of William of Brescia)." *Sudhoffs Archiv* (1972): 113–44.

– "Chemical Medicine in the Medical Writings of Arnau de Vilanova." *Arxiu de textos catalans antics* (2005): 239–67.

– "Theriac at Montpellier 1285–1325 (with an edition of the 'Questiones de tyriaca' of William of Brescia)." *Sudhoffs Archiv* (1972): 113–44.

Mel'gunov, S.P., "Iz istorii vrachebnago i aptechnago dela v Rossii. (Istoricheskaia spravka po povodu 200-letiia ucherezhdeniia vol'nykh aptek)." *Farmatsevticheskii vestnik* 8 (1901): 95–7.

Mendoza, Ruben G., and Jay R. Wolter. "Medicine in Meso and South America." In *Encyclopaedia of the History of Science, Technology and Medicine in Non-Western Cultures*, ed. Helaine Selin, 702–06. Dortrecht: Springer Science + Business Media, 1997.

Mikhailov, S.S. *Meditsinskaia sluzhba russkogo flota v XVIII veke. Materialy k istorii otechestvennoj meditsiny*. Medgiz: Leningrad, 1957.

Mil'kov, V.V. "Antichnoe uchenie o chetyrekh stikhiiakh v drevnerusskoi pis'mennosti." In *Drevniaia Rus': Peresechenie traditsii*, ed. V.V. Mil'kov, M.Iu. Neborskii, C.V. Mil'kov, and G.S. Barankova, 57–66. Moscow: NITs "Skriptorii," 1997.

Miller, David. "The Lübeckers Bartholomaeus Ghotan and Nicolaus Bülow in Novgorod and Moscow and the Problem of Early Western Influences on Russian Culture." *Viator. Medieval and Renaissance Studies* 9 (1978): 395–412.

Mirksii, M. B., "Aptekarskii prikaz (k 410-letiiu gosudarstvennogo upravleniia meditsinskimi delami v Rossii)." *Sovetskoe zdravookhranenie* 11 (1991): 72–7.

– *Meditsina Rossii XVI–XIX vekov*. Moscow: ROSSPEN, 1996.

– *Meditsina Rossii X–XX vekov. Ocherki istorii*. Moscow: ROSSPEN, 2005.

Monahan, Erika. "Locating Rhubarb: Early Modernity's Relevant Obscurity." In *Early Modern Things: Objects and Their Histories, 1500–1800*, ed. Paula Findlen, 227–51. London and New York: Routledge, 2013.

– *The Merchants of Siberia: Trade in Early Modern Eurasia*. Ithaca, NY: Cornell University Press, 2016.

Moran, Bruce T. "A Survey of Chemical Medicine in the 17th Century: Spanning Court, Classroom, and Cultures." *Pharmacy in History* 38, no. 3 (1996): 121–33.

Morozov, B.N. "Posleslovie 1616g. k travniku Liubchanina – zabytyi istochnik po istorii knizhnykh sobranii russkikh tsarei XVI-nachala XVII v." *Istochnikovedenie i kraevedenie v kul'ture Rossii* (2000): 131–5.

– "K istorii Travnika Liubchanina 1533/34g." *Arkheograficheskii ezhegodnik za 2000 god*, 112–14. Moscow: Nauka, 2001.

– "Travnik iz Postel'noi kazny Ivana Groznogo? Khar'kovskaia rukopis'

1534g. – novyi pamiatnik knizhnoi masterskoi mitropolita Daniila (Pervye itogi izucheniia)." *Arkheograficheskii ezhegodnik za 2002 god*, 73–85. Moscow: Nauka, 2004.

– "Vertograd zdraviiu: Travnik iz biblioteki Ivana Groznogo." *Rodina* (2004): 36–40.

– "Novoe o travnike 1616g. (Parizhskaia nakhodka)." *Vospomogatel'nye istoricheskie distsipliny: klassicheskoe nasledie i novye napravleniia* (2006): 314–16.

Morozov, B.N., and R.A. Simonov. "Datirovka i atributsiia mediko-astrologicheskikh raschetov, pripisannykh k Travniky 1534 goda." *Drevniaia Rus' Voprosy Medievistiki* 4 (2004): 5–21.

Morozov, N.N. "Po povodu organizatsii pervoi apteki," *Aptechnoe delo* 6 (1952): 47–50.

Mukharji, Projit Bihari. *Doctoring Traditions: Ayurveda, Small Technologies, and Braided Sciences*. Chicago: University of Chicago Press, 2016.

Muskala, Johan. "K tekstologii Travnika Liubchanina (nekotorye nabliudeniia)." In *I.I. Sreznevskii i russkoe istoricheskoe iazykoznanie: K 200–letiiu so dnia rozhdeniia I.I. Sreznevskogo*, ed. I.M. Sheina and O.V. Nikitin, 258–67. Riazan': Riazanskii gosudarstvennyi universitet im. S.A, Esenina, 2012.

Nanzatov B.Z., and M.M. Sodnompilova. "Lekarstvennye sredstva v torgovo-obmennykh operatsiiakh mezhdu Rossiei, Mongoliei i Kitaem v XVII–XIX vv." *Vestnik nauchnogo tsentra Sibirskogo otdeleniia Rossiiskoi akademii nauk* 4, no. 16 (2014): 90–8.

Nappi, Carla. "Bolatu's Pharmacy: Theriac in Early Modern China." *Early Science and Medicine* 14, no. 6 (2009): 737–64.

– *The Monkey and the Inkpot: Natural History and Its Transformations in Early Modern China*. Cambridge: Harvard University Press, 2010.

– "Surface Tension: Objectifying Ginseng in Chinese Early Modernity." In *Early Modern Things: Objects and Their Histories, 1500–1800*, ed. Paula Findlen, 31–52. Abingdon: Routledge, 2013.

Neilson, Brett, and Mohammed Bamyeh. "Drugs in Motion: Toward a Materialist Tracking of Global Mobilities." *Cultural Critique* 71, no. 1 (2009): 1–12.

New Revised Standard Version Bible. Anglicised Edition. Oxford: Oxford University Press, 1995.

Newman, William, and Lawrence Principe. *Alchemy Tried in the Fire: Starkey, Boyle, and The Fate of Helmontian Chymistry*. Chicago: University of Chicago Press, 2005.

Newson, Linda A. *Making Medicines in Early Colonial Lima, Peru: Apothecaries, Science and Society*. Leiden: Brill, 2017.

Norton, Marcy. "Tasting Empire: Chocolate and the European Internalization of Mesoamerican Aesthetics." *American Historical Review* 111, no. 3 (2006): 660–91.

– *Sacred Gifts, Profane Pleasures: A History of Tobacco and Chocolate in the Atlantic World.* Ithaca: Cornell University Press 2008.

Novombergskii, N.Ia. *Ocherki po istorii aptechnago dela v do-Petrovskoi Rusi.* St Petersburg: Tipografiia Ministerstva Vnutrennikh del, 1902.

– *Materialy po istorii meditsiny v Rossii.* 5 vols. St Petersburg: M.M. Stasiulevich, 1905.

– *Vrachebnoe stroenie v do-Petrovskoi Rusi.* Tomsk: Parovaia tipolitografiia Sibirskogo tovarishchestva pechatnogo dela, 1907.

Nutton, Vivian "What's in an Oath?" *Journal of the Royal College of Physicians of London* 29, no. 6 (1995): 518–24.

Okenfuss, Max J. *The Rise and Fall of Latin Humanism in Early-Modern Russia. Pagan Authors, Ukrainians, and the Resiliency of Muscovy.* Leiden, New York, Cologne: E.J. Brill, 1995.

Oparina, T.A. *Inozemtsy v Rossii XVI–XVII vv.* Moscow: Progress-Traditsiia, 2007.

"Opis' domashnemu imushchestvu tsaria Ivana Vasilevicha po spiskam 90 i 91 godov." *Vremennik Imperatorskogo Moskovskogo obshchestva istorii i drevnostei rossiiskikh* 7. Moscow: Universitetskaia typografiia, 1850.

Opyt istoricheskogo ocherka voznikovenie i razvitiia vsego aptekarskogo dela v Rossii, a v chastnosti staroi Nikolskoi apteki prinadlezhashchei nyne Tovarishchestvu "V.K. Ferrein" i osnovannoi v 1701 godu v tsarstvovanie Imperatora Petra Velikago, Daniilom Gurchinym. Moscow: Tipo-Litografiia Tovarishchestva I.N. Kushnerev, 1911.

Oreshnikov, A.V. "Danil Gurchin. Moskovskii aptekar' nachala XVIII veka." In *Sbornik statei v chest' grafini Praskov'i Sergeevny Uvarovoi*, 47–69. Moscow: [n. pub.], 1916.

Orlenko, S.P. *Vykhodtsy iz zapadnoi Evropy v Rossii XVII veka. Pravovoi status i real'noe polozhenie.* Moscow: Drevlekhranilishche, 2004.

Panich, T.V. *Literaturnoe tvorchestvo Afanasiia Kholmogorskogo.* Novosibirsk: Sibirskii khronograf, 1996.

Panova, T.D. *Kremlevskie usypal'nitsy. Istoriya, sud'ba, taina.* Moscow: Indrik, 2003.

Pantin, Isabelle. "The Role of Translations in European Scientific Exchanges in the Sixteenth and Seventeenth Centuries." In *Cultural Translation in Early Modern Europe*, ed. Peter Burke and R. Po-Chia Hsia, 163–79. Cambridge: Cambridge University Press, 2007.

Parascandola, John. *King of Poisons: A History of Arsenic*. Washington, DC: Potomac Books, 2012.

Pareja, Francisco. *Confessionario en lengua Castellana y Timuquana con unos consejos para animar al penitente. Y assi mismo van declarados algunos effectos y prerrogariuas deste sancto sacramento de la Confession. Todo muy util y prouechoso, assi para que los padres confessores sepan instruyr al penitente como para que ellos aprendan à saber se confessar*. Mexico, 1613. http://www.archive.org/stream/confessionarioenoopare (accessed 9 September 2019).

Park, Katharine. "The Life of the Corpse: Division and Dissection in Late Medieval Europe." *Journal of the History of Medicine and Allied Sciences* 50, no. 1 (1995): 111–32.

Pavlov, A.P., "Prikazy i prikaznaia biurokratiia (1584–1605 gg.)." *Istoricheskie zapiski* 116 (1988): 187–227.

Pelling, Margaret. *The Common Lot: Sickness, Medical Occupations and the Urban Poor in Early Modern England*. New York: Routledge, 2014.

Pelling, Margaret, and Frances White. *Medical Conflicts in Early Modern London: Patronage, Physicians, and Irregular Practitioners, 1550–1640*. Oxford: Oxford University Press, 2003.

Petrov, Avvakum. *Zhitie Protopopa Avvakuma, im samim napisannoe*. Moscow and Augsburg: Werden Verlag, 2003.

Pickwoad, Nicholas, "Bookbinding." In *Companion to the History of the Book*, vol. 1, ed. Simon Eliot and Jonathan Rose, 111–27. Hoboken: John Wiley & Sons, 2020.

Plavsic, Borivoj. "Seventeenth-Century Chanceries and Their Staffs." In *Russian Officialdom: The Bureaucratization of Russian Society from the Seventeenth to the Twentieth Century*, ed. Walter McKenzie Pintner and Don Karl Rowney, 19–45. London: Macmillan, 1980.

Pluskowski, Aleksander. "Narwhals or Unicorns? Exotic Animals as Material Culture in Medieval Europe." *European Journal of Archaeology* 7, no. 3 (2004): 291–313.

Poe, Marshall T. "Tsar Aleksei Mikhailovich and the End of the Romanov Political Settlement." *Russian Review* 62 (2003): 537–64.

Poe, Marshall T. ed. *Samuel Collins. The Present State of Russia In a Letter to a Friend at London: Written by an Eminent Person residing at the Great Czars Court at Mosco for the space of nine years. [London, 1671; from the first edi-*

tion at Houghton Library, Harvard University]. Iowa Research Online, 2008. https://iro.uiowa.edu/discovery/delivery/01IOWA_INST:ResearchRepository/12674991920002771?l#13675491870002771.

Polnoe sobanie zakonov Rossisskoi Imperii. Sobranie pervoe. 1649–1825. 45 vols. St Petersburg: Tip II otdeleniia sobstvennoi ego imperatorskogo velichestva kantseliarii, 1830.

Porter, Roy. *The Greatest Benefit to Mankind: A Medical History of Humanity from Antiquity to the Present*. London: HarperCollins, 1997.

Prozorovskii, V.I., I.V. Alisievich, E.I Kanter, and A.F. Rubtsov. "Issledovanie ostatkov tsaria Ivana IV, ego sinovei i kniazia Skopina-Shuiskogo." *Sudebno-meditsinskaia ekspertiza* 12, no. 1 (1969): 19–21.

Prozorovskii, V.I., and V.M. Kolosova. "Nekotorye dannye isledovaniia spektral'nym metodom kostnoi tkani tsaria Ivana IV, ego sinovei i kniazia Skopina-Shuiskogo." *Sudebno-meditsinskaia ekspertiza* 13, no. 2 (1970): 7–11.

Prussak, A.B. "Iz istorii aptechnogo dela na Rusi." *Aptechnoe delo* 6 (1953): 56–9.

– "Obzor meditsinskikh rukopisei XVII–XVIII vv., khraniaschikhsia v Leningradskoi gosudarstvennoi Publichnoi biblioteke im. Saltykova-Shchedrina, kak istochnika po istorii primeneniia lekarstvennykh rastenii." RNL, f. 1000, op. 2, ed. khr. 1123, 1954: 24–5.

Pugliano, Valentina. "Botanical Artisans: Apothecaries and the Study of Nature in Venice and London, 1550–1610." Unpublished PhD diss., University of Oxford, 2013.

– "Specimen Lists: Artisanal Writing or Natural Historical Paperwork?" *Isis* 103, no. 4 (2012): 716–26.

– "Pharmacy, Testing, and the Language of Truth in Renaissance Italy." *Bulletin of the History of Medicine* 91, no. 2 (2017): 233–73.

Quincy, John. *Pharmacopoeia Officinalis & Extemporanea: Or a Compleat English Dispensatory*. London: Printed for T. Longman, 1719.

Raj, Kapil. *Relocating Modern Science: Circulation and the Construction of Knowledge in South Asia and Europe 1650–1900*. New York: Palgrave Macmillan, 2007.

– "Beyond Postcolonialism … and Postpositivism: Circulation and the Global History of Science." *Isis* 104, no. 2 (2013): 337–47.

Rankin, Alisha. "Empirics, Physicians, and Wonder Drugs in Early Modern Germany: The Case of the Panacea Amwaldina." *Early Science and Medicine* 14, no. 6 (2009): 680–710.

– "On Anecdote and Antidotes: Poison Trials in Sixteenth-Century Europe." *Bulletin of the History of Medicine* 91, no. 2 (2017): 274–302.

– *The Poison Trials: Wonder Drugs, Experiment, and the Battle for Authority in Renaissance Science*. Chicago: University of Chicago Press, 2021.

Renner, Andreas. "Wissenschaftstransfer ins zarenreich des 18. Jahrhunderts. Bemerkungen zum forschungsstand am beispiel der medizingeschichte." *Jahrbücher für Geschichte Osteuropas* H. 1 (2005): 64–85.

– *Russische Autokratie und europäische Medizin. Organisierter Wissenstransfer im 18 Jahrhundert*. Stuttgart: Franz Steiner, 2010.

Richter, Wilhelm. *Geschichte der medicin in Russland*. Moscow: N.S. Vsevoloski, 1813–17.

Romaniello, Matthew P. "Muscovy's Extraordinary Ban on Tobacco." In *Tobacco in Russian History and Culture*, ed. Matthew P. Romaniello and Tricia Starks, 19–35. London: Routledge, 2011.

– "Humoral Bodies in Cold Climates." In *Russian History through the Senses: From 1700 to the Present*, ed. Matthew P. Romaniello and Tricia Starks, 23–43. London: Bloomsbury Publishing, 2016.

– "True Rhubarb? Trading Eurasian Botanical and Medical Knowledge in the Eighteenth Century." *Journal of Global History* 11, no. 1 (2016): 3–23.

Rowell, Margery. "Russian Medical Botany before the Time of Peter the Great." *Sudhoffs Archiv* 62 (1978): 339–58.

Rowland, Daniel. "The Problem of Advice in Muscovite Tales about the Time of Troubles." *Russian History* 6, no. 2 (1979): 259–83.

Ryan, William F. "The Old Russian Version of the Pseudo-Aristotelian '*Secreta Secretorum*.'" *Slavonic and East European Review* 56, no. 2 (1978): 242–60.

– "The *Secretum Secretorum* and the Muscovite Autocracy." In *Pseudo-Aristotle: The* Secret of Secrets*: Sources and Influences*, ed. William F. Ryan and Charles B. Schmidt, 114–23. London: Warburg Institute Surveys, 1982.

– "Alchemy, Magic, Poisons and the Virtues of Stones in the Old Russian *Secretum Secretorum*." *Ambix* 37, no. 1 (1990): 46–54.

– "Alchemy and the Virtues of Stones in Muscovy." In *Alchemy and Chemistry in the 16th and 17th Centuries*, ed. Piyo Rattansi and Antonio Clericuzio, 149–59. Dordrecht: Klewer Academic Publishers, 1994.

– *The Bathhouse at Midnight: An Historical Survey of Magic and Divination in Russia*. University Park: Pennsylvania State University Press, 1999.

Rybalko, N.V. *Rossiiskaia prikaznaia biurokratiia v Smutnoe Vremia nachala XVII v.* Moscow: Kvadriga, 2011.

Savage-Smith, Emilie. "Drug Therapy of Eye Diseases in Seventeenth-Century Islamic Medicine: The Influence of the 'New Chemistry' of the Paracelsians." *Pharmacy in History* 29, no. 1 (1987): 3–28.

Savel'eva, E.A. *Katalog knig iz sobraniia Aptekarskogo prikaza*. St Petersburg: Alfaret, 2006.

Saxer, Martin. "Tibetan Medicine and Russian Modernities." In *Medicine between Science and Religion: Explorations on Tibetan Grounds*, ed. Vincanne Adams, Mona Schrempf, and Sienna R. Craig, 57–82. New York: Berghahn, 2010.

Scheper, Karin. *The Technique of Islamic Bookbinding: Methods, Materials and Regional Varieties*. Leiden: Brill, 2018.

Schiebinger, Londa. "Feminist History of Colonial Science." *Hypatia* 19, no. 1 (2004): 233–54.

Schilling, Ruth, Sabine Schlegelmilch, and Susan Splinter. "Stadtarzt oder Arzt in der Stadt? Drei Ärzte der Frühen Neuzeit und ihr Verständnis des städtischen Amtes." *Medizinhistorisches Journal* 46, no. 2 (2011): 99–133.

Schmitz-Esser, Romedio. *Der Leichnam im Mittelalter. Einbalsamierung, Verbrennung und die kulturelle Konstruktion des toten Körpers*. Ostfildern: Jan Thorbecke, 2014.

Schröder, Johann, *Pharmocopoeia medicochymica siue Thesaurus Pharmocologius, quo Composita quaque Celebriore; Hinc mineralia, vegilabilia et animalia chymico-medice, describuntur, atque ni super Principia physica Hermetico Hypocratia candide exhibentur*. 1600–64.

Shapin, Steven. "The Invisible Technician." *American Scientist* 77, no. 6 (1989): 554–63.

Shaw, James, and Evelyn Welch. *Making and Marketing Medicine in Renaissance Florence*. Leiden: Brill, 2011.

Shefer-Mossensohn, Miri. *Ottoman Medicine: Healing and Medical Institutions, 1500–1700*. Albany: SUNY Press, 2010.

Shepard, Odell. *The Lore of the Unicorn. Myths and Legends*. London: G. Allen and Unwin, 1930; London: Senate, 1996.

Shevyrev, Stepan Petrovich. "Vvedenie v istoriiu russkoi slovesnosti. Chtenie pervoe," *Moskvitianin*, 1844 no. 1. 219–40; no. 2, 534–59; no. 3, 118–39; no. 4, 305–24; no. 8, 285–317.

Shkunov, V.N. "Aptekarskii prikaz i vneshniaia torgovlia Rossii v XVII–nachale XVIII vv." *Moskovskoe obozrenie* 6 (2011): 2–3.

Shmidt, S.O., and S.E. Kniaz'kov. *Dokumenty deloproizvodstva pravitel'stvennykh uchrezhdenii Rossii XVI–XVII vv. Uchebnoe posobie*. Moscow: MGIAI, 1985.

Sibirtsaev, Mikhail. *Opyt Bibleisko-estestvennoi istorii, ili opisatel'noe izlozhenie Bibleiskoi geologii, botaniki i zoologii*, 252–6. St Petersburg: Strannik, 1897.

Simioli, Carmen. "The King of Essences: Mercury in the Tibetan Medicoalchemical Traditions." A.I.O.N.: *annali dell'Istituto Universitario Orientale di Napoli: Dipartimento di studi del mondo classico e del Mediterraneoantico antico: sezione filologico-letteraria: XXXVII* (2015): 35–54.

Simonov, R.A. "Rossiiskie pridvornye 'matimatiki' XVI–XVII vekov." *Voprosy istorii* 1 (1986): 76–83.

– *Russkaia astrologicheskaia knizhnost' (XI–pervaia chetvert' XVIII veka).* Moscow: Izdatel'stvo MGUP "Mir knigi," 1998.

Siraisi, Nancy. *History, Medicine, and the Traditions of Renaissance Learning.* Ann Arbor: University of Michigan Press, 2007.

Sivasundaram, Sujit, et al. "Global Histories of Science." Special section of *Isis* 101 (2010).

Skrynnikov, R.G. *Tsarstvo terrora.* St Petersburg: Nauka, 1992.

Slater, John, Maríaluz López-Terrada, and José Pardo-Tomás, eds. *Medical Cultures of the Early Modern Spanish Empire.* New York: Routledge, 2016.

Slukhovskii, M. I., *Bibliotechnoe delo v Rossii do XVII veka. Iz istorii knizhnogo prosviashcheniia.* Moscow: Kniga, 1968.

Smilianskaia, E.B., *Volshebniki, bogokhul'niki, eretiki: narodnaia religioznost' i "dukhovnye prestupleniia" v Rossii XVIII v.* Moskva: Indrik, 2003.

Smith, Pamela H. *The Body of the Artisan: Art and Experience in the Scientific Revolution.* Chicago: University of Chicago Press, 2018.

– ed. *Entangled Itineraries: Materials, Practices, and Knowledges across Eurasia.* Pittsburgh: University of Pittsburgh Press, 2019.

Smith, Pamela H., Amy R.W. Meyers, and Harold J. Cook, eds. *Ways of Making and Knowing: The Material Culture of Empirical Knowledge.* Ann Arbor: University of Michigan Press, 2017.

Smith-Peter, Susan. "Russian America in Russian and American Historiography." *Kritika: Explorations in Russian and Eurasian History* 14, no. 1 (2013): 93–100.

Sobranie gosudarstvennykh gramot i dogovorov, khraniashchikhsia v gosudarstvennoi kollegii inostrannykh del. 4 vols. Moscow: Tip. N.S. Vsevolozhskii, 1813–1826.

Sokolovskii, M.K. "Kharakter i znachenie deiatel'nosti Aptekarskogo prikaza." *Vestnik arkheologii i istorii* 16 (1904): 60–89.

Song, Minah. "The History and Characteristics of Traditional Korean Books and Bookbinding." *Journal of the Institute of Conservation* 32, no. 1 (2009): 53–78.

Spary, Emma C. *Eating the Enlightenment: Food and the Sciences in Paris, 1670–1760.* Chicago: University of Chicago Press, 2013.

– "On the Ironic Specimen of the Unicorn Horn in Enlightened Cabinets." *Journal of Social History* 52, no. 4 (2019): 1033–60.

Stenfors, Jenifer L., and Richard Hellie. "The Elite Clergy Diet in Late Muscovy." *Russian History* 22 (1995): 1–23.

Stephenson, Marcia. "From Marvelous Antidote to the Poison of Idolatry: The Transatlantic Role of Andean Bezoar Stones during the Late Sixteenth and Early Seventeenth Centuries." *Hispanic American Historical Review* 90, no. 1 (2010): 3–39.

Stolberg, Michael. "'Abhorreas pinguedinem': Fat and Obesity in Early Modern Medicine (c. 1500–1750)." *Studies in History and Philosophy of Biological and Biomedical Sciences* 43 (2012): 370–8.

Stoliarova, L.V., and S.M. Kashtanov. *Kniga v drevnei Rusi (XI–XVI vv.).* Moscow: Universitet Dmitriia Pozharskogo, 2010.

Stone, Gerald, *A Dictionarie of the Vulgar Russe Tongue, Attributed to Mark Ridley, Edited from the late-sixteenth-century manuscripts and with an introduction.* Köln, Weimar, Wien: Böhlau Verlag, 1996.

Sugg, Richard. "'Good Physic but Bad Food': Early Modern Attitudes to Medicinal Cannibalism and Its Suppliers." *Social History of Medicine* 19, no. 2 (2006): 225–40.

– *Mummies, Cannibals, and Vampires: The History of Corpse Medicine from the Renaissance to the Victorians.* London and New York: Routledge, 2011.

Thyrêt, Isolde. "'Blessed Is the Tsaritsa's Womb': The Myth of Miraculous Birth and Royal Motherhood in Muscovite Russia." *Russian Review* 53, no. 4 (1994): 479–96.

Tkeshelashvili, I.S. *Russkaia farmatsiia do voznikoveniia pervykh volnykh aptek v Rossii.* Moscow: Tipo-litografiia I. N. Kushnerev, 1902.

– *Prakticheskoe rukovodstvo vrachei i farmatsevtov.* Moscow: Tipografiia Russkogo Tovarishchstva pechatnogo i izdaltel'stvago dela, 1905.

Trambaiolo, Daniel. "Antisyphilitic Mercury Drugs in Early Modern China and Japan." *Asiatische Studien-Études Asiatiques* 69, no. 4 (2015): 997–1016.

Treue, Wolfgang. "Lebensbedingungen jüdischer Ärzte in Frankfurt am Main während des Spätmittelalters und der Frühen Neuzeit." *Medizin, Gesellschaft und Geschichte. Jahrbuch des Instituts für Geschichte der Medizin der Robert Bosch Stiftung, Bd* 17 (2015): 9–55.

Tsvataev, D.V. *Protestantskie tserkvi i dukhovenstvo. Iz istorii inostrannykh ispovedanii v Rossii v XVI i XVII vekakh.* Moscow: Universitetskaia tipografiia, 1866.

– *Mediki v Moskovskoi Rossii i pervyi russkii doktor. Istoriko-biograficheskii ocherk.* Varshava: Tipografiia Varshavskogo instituta glukhonemykh i slepykh, 1896.

Unkovskaya, Maria. "Learning Foreign Mysteries: Russian Pupils of the Aptekarskii Prikaz, 1650–1700." *Oxford Slavonic Papers* 30 (1997): 1–20.

– *Brief Lives: A Handbook of Medical Practitioners in Muscovy, 1620–1701.* London: Wellcome Trust, 1999.

Ustiugov, N.V., "Evoliutsiia prikaznogo stroia russkogo gosudarstva v XVII v." In *Absoliutizm v Rossii XVII–XVIII vv: Sbornik statei k semidesiatiletiiu so dnia rozhdeniia i sorokapiatiletiiu nauchnoi i pedagogicheskoi deiatel'nosti B. B. Kafengauza*, ed. N. M. Druzhinin, 134–67. Moscow: Nauka, 1964.

Utkin, L.A. *Kratkii botanicheskii russko-latinskii slovar'*. Moscow: Akademii nauk SSSR, 1962.

Veluwenkamp, Jan Willem, and Werner Scheltjens. "Baltic Drugs Traffic, 1650–1850. Sound Toll Registers Online as a Source for the Import of Exotic Medicines in the Baltic Sea Area." *Social History of Medicine* 31, no. 1 (2018): 140–76.

Viktorov, A. *Sobranie slaviano-russkikh rukopisei V.M. Undolskogo. Bibliograficheskii ocherk.* Moscow: Universitetskaia tipografiia, 1870.

Vinkovetsky, Ilya. *Russian America: An Overseas Colony of a Continental Empire, 1804–1867*. Oxford: Oxford University Press, 2011.

Walker, Timothy. "The Early Modern Globalization of Indian Medicine: Portuguese Dissemination of Drugs and Healing Techniques from South Asia on Four Continents, 1670–1830." *Portuguese Literary and Cultural Studies* 17/18 (2010): 77–97.

Wallis, Patrick. "Exotic Drugs and English Medicine: England's Drug Trade, c. 1550–c. 1800." *Social History of Medicine* 25, no. 1 (2011): 20–46.

Watson, Christine. *Tradition and Translation: Maciej Stryjkowski's Polish Chronicle in Seventeenth-Century Russian Manuscripts.* Upsala: Acta Universitatis Upsaliensis, 2012.

Waugh, Daniel Clarke. "The Unsolved Problem of Tsar Ivan IV's Library." *Russian History* 14, no. 1 (1987): 395–408.

Weickhardt, George G. "Bureaucrats and Boiars in the Muscovite Tsardom." *Russian History* 10, no. 3 (1983): 342–9.

Wendt, Helge, ed. *The Globalization of Knowledge in the Iberian Colonial World*. Berlin: Max Planck Research Library, 2016.

Werrett, Simon. *Fireworks: Pyrotechnic Arts and Sciences in European History*. Chicago: University of Chicago Press, 2010.

Winterbottom, Anna E. "Of the China Root: A Case Study of the Early Modern Circulation of Materia Medica." *Social History of Medicine* 28, no. 1 (2014): 22–44.

Wittop Koning, D.A. *Compendium voor de geschiedenis van de pharmacie van Nederland* Lochem: De Tijdstrom, 1986.

Woodall, John. *The Surgions Mate.* London, 1617.

Yoder, Audra Jo. "Tea Time in Romanov Russia: A Cultural History, 1616–1917." Unpublished PhD diss., University of North Carolina at Chapel Hill, 2016.

Zabivkin, I. "Travnik." *Olonetskaia nedelia* 17 (1911): 12–14.

Zagoskin, N.P., *Vrachi i vrachebnoe delo v starinnoi Rossii.* Kazan: Tip. Imperatorskogo Universiteta, 1891.

Zakharov, V.N. *Zapadnoevropeiskie kuptsy v rossiiskom torgovle XVIII veka.* Moscow: Nauka, 2005.

Zapasko, Ia.P. *Pam'iatki knizhkovogo mistetstva. Ukrains'ka rukopisna kniga.* Lviv: Svit, 1995.

Zarubin, N.N. *Biblioteka Ivana Groznogo. Rekonstruktiia i bibliograficheskoe opisanie.* Leningrad: Nauka, 1982.

Zharinov, G.V. "Zapisi o Raskhode Lekarstvennykh Sredstv 1581–1582gg." *Arkhiv Russkoi istorii. Nauchnyi istoricheskii zhurnal* 4 (1994): 103–24.

Zhinkin, N.P., "Kratkie svedeniia o rukopisiakh Tsentral'noi nauchnoi biblioteki Khar'kovskogo gosudarstvennogo universiteta im. A.M. Gor'kogo." In *Trudy Otdela drevenrusskoi literatury Instituta russkoi literatury (Pushkinskogo doma)* AN SSSR IX, 467–75. Moscow and Leningrad: Izdatel'tsvo AN SSSR, 1953.

Zitser, Ernest A. *The Transfigured Kingdom: Sacred Parody and Charismatic Authority at the Court of Peter the Great.* Ithaca: Cornell University Press, 2018.

Zmeev, L.F., *Russkie vrachebniki. Issledovanie v oblasti nashei drevnei vrachebnoi pis'mennosti,* Pamiatniki drevnei pis'mennosti i iskustva, no. 112 (St Petersburg: [n. pub.], 1896).

Index

www.ingramcontent.com/pod-product-compliance
Lightning Source LLC
LaVergne TN
LVHW040601130826
845408LV00028B/302